Future Research Needs Paper

I0470819

Number 24

PCA3 Testing in the Diagnosis and Management of Prostate Cancer: Future Research Needs

Identification of Future Research Needs From Comparative Effectiveness Review No. 98

Prepared for:
Agency for Healthcare Research and Quality
U.S. Department of Health and Human Services
540 Gaither Road
Rockville, MD 20850
www.ahrq.gov

Contract No. 290-2007-10058-I

Prepared by:
Blue Cross and Blue Shield Association Technology Evaluation Center Evidence-based Practice Center
Chicago, IL

Investigators:
Steven I. Gutman, M.D., M.B.A.
Denise M. Oliansky, M.A., M.L.I.S.
Suzanne Belinson, Ph.D., M.P.H.
Naomi Aronson, Ph.D.

AHRQ Publication No. 13-EHC005-EF
April 2013

This report is based on research conducted by the Blue Cross and Blue Shield Association Technology Evaluation Center Evidence-based Practice Center (EPC) under contract to the Agency for Healthcare Research and Quality (AHRQ), Rockville, MD (Contract No. 290-2007-10058-I). The findings and conclusions in this document are those of the author(s), who are responsible for its contents; the findings and conclusions do not necessarily represent the views of AHRQ. Therefore, no statement in this report should be construed as an official position of AHRQ or of the U.S. Department of Health and Human Services.

The information in this report is intended to help health care researchers and funders of research make well-informed decisions in designing and funding research and thereby improve the quality of health care services. This report is not intended to be a substitute for the application of scientific judgment. Anyone who makes decisions concerning the provision of clinical care should consider this report in the same way as any medical research and in conjunction with all other pertinent information, i.e., in the context of available resources and circumstances.

This document is in the public domain and may be used and reprinted without special permission. Citation of the source is appreciated.

Persons using assistive technology may not be able to fully access information in this report. For assistance contact EffectiveHealthCare@ahrq.hhs.gov.

Suggested citation: Gutman SI, Oliansky DM, Belinson S, Aronson N. PCA3 Testing in the Diagnosis and Management of Prostate Cancer: Future Research Needs. Future Research Needs Paper No. 24. (Prepared by the Blue Cross and Blue Shield Association Technology Evaluation Center Evidence-based Practice Center under Contract No. 290-2007-10058-I.) AHRQ Publication No. 13-EHC005-EF. Rockville, MD: Agency for Healthcare Research and Quality. April 2013. www.effectivehealthcare.ahrq.gov/reports/final.cfm.

Preface

The Agency for Healthcare Research and Quality (AHRQ), through its Evidence-based Practice Centers (EPCs), sponsors the development of evidence reports and technology assessments to assist public- and private-sector organizations in their efforts to improve the quality of health care in the United States. The reports and assessments provide organizations with comprehensive, science-based information on common, costly medical conditions and new health care technologies and strategies. The EPCs systematically review the relevant scientific literature on topics assigned to them by AHRQ and conduct additional analyses when appropriate prior to developing their reports and assessments.

An important part of evidence reports is to not only synthesize the evidence, but also to identify the gaps in evidence that limited the ability to answer the systematic review questions. AHRQ supports EPCs to work with various stakeholders to identify and prioritize the future research that is needed by decisionmakers. This information is provided for researchers and funders of research in these Future Research Needs papers. These papers are made available for public comment and use and may be revised.

AHRQ expects that the EPC evidence reports and technology assessments will inform individual health plans, providers, and purchasers as well as the health care system as a whole by providing important information to help improve health care quality. The evidence reports undergo public comment prior to their release as a final report.

We welcome comments on this Future Research Needs document. They may be sent by mail to the Task Order Officer named below at: Agency for Healthcare Research and Quality, 540 Gaither Road, Rockville, MD 20850, or by email to epc@ahrq.hhs.gov.

Carolyn M. Clancy, M.D.
Director
Agency for Healthcare Research and Quality

Jean Slutsky, P.A., M.S.P.H
Director, Center for Outcomes and Evidence
Agency for Healthcare Research and Quality

Stephanie Chang, M.D., M.P.H.
Director, EPC Program
Center for Outcomes and Evidence
Agency for Healthcare Research and Quality

Supriya Janakiraman, M.D., M.P.H.
Task Order Officer
Center for Outcomes and Evidence
Agency for Healthcare Research and Quality

Acknowledgments

The Research Team would like to acknowledge the following individuals for their contributions to this report: Hussein Noorani, M.S.; Glenn Palomaki, Ph.D.; Linda A. Bradley, Ph.D., FACMG; Elaine Alligood, M.L.S.; Lisa Sarsany, M.A.; Lisa Garofalo, B.A.; and Kathleen M. Ziegler, Pharm.D.

Stakeholder Panel

The following individuals served as members of the Stakeholder Panel described in this report. Broad expertise and perspectives are sought and their contributions were invaluable. Divergent and conflicted opinions are common and perceived as healthy scientific discourse. Therefore, in the end, study questions, design, and/or methodologic approaches do not necessarily represent the views of individual technical and content experts.

Todd Alonzo, Ph.D.
University of Southern California
Arcadia, CA

Robert Carey, B.S.
Georgia Prostate Cancer Coalition/Georgia
  Ovarian Cancer Alliance
Atlanta, GA

W. David Dotson, Ph.D.
Centers for Disease Control and Prevention
Atlanta, GA

John L. Gore, M.D., M.S.
University of Washington
Seattle, WA

Roger Klein, M.D., J.D.
Blood Center of Wisconsin
Milwaukee, WI

Howard Parnes, M.D.
Division of Cancer Prevention
National Cancer Institute
Bethesda, MD

Richard Rainey, M.D.
Regence BlueShield of Idaho
Lewiston, ID

Andrew Stephenson, M.D.
Center for Urologic Oncology
Cleveland Clinic
Cleveland, OH

PCA3 Testing in the Diagnosis and Management of Prostate Cancer: Future Research Needs

Structured Abstract

Background. Cancer of the prostate is the second most common cancer and the second leading cause of cancer deaths in men in the United States. Screening to detect disease using the total prostate-specific antigen test is a common but controversial practice. The prostate cancer antigen-3 gene (PCA3) has recently been found to be overexpressed in prostate cancers, is measurable in urine, and may be a useful biomarker for improving the results of cancer screening programs.

Objectives. The objective of this report was to generate prioritized topics for future research on PCA3, building on evidence gaps identified in a prior draft Comparative Effectiveness Review (CER) and following an explicit stakeholder-driven nomination and prioritization process.

Data sources. Data sources included a draft CER on PCA3, a comprehensive literature search, and input from members of the Stakeholder Panel.

Methods. Building on evidence gaps identified in a draft CER on PCA3, a preliminary list of future research needs was developed. This was reviewed and refined using input from a diverse group of stakeholders with a common interest in prostate cancer. Stakeholders were asked to prioritize topics using the following elements: current importance, potential for significant health impact, incremental value, and feasibility. An iterative process, including the use of teleconferences and SurveyMonkey®, an online survey tool, was used to prioritize research needs and questions.

Results. Three high-priority research needs were identified, as well as seven research questions. These included the need for information on the comparative performance of PCA3 versus currently used prostate cancer biomarkers, studies on how PCA3 affects biopsy decisionmaking, and studies on how PCA3 affects long-term health outcomes.

Conclusions. A variety of future research needs were identified and prioritized to inform future study of PCA3. This research should help to determine the role PCA3 should play in the diagnosis and management of patients with prostate cancer.

Contents

Appendixes

Executive Summary

Background

Cancer of the prostate is the second most common cancer and the second leading cause of cancer deaths in men in the United States.[1] Most patients have indolent tumors and may live for years with no or minimal effects, ultimately dying of other causes.[2] However, some patients have aggressive tumors that spread beyond the prostate, resulting in significant morbidity and death.

The rationale for prostate cancer screening using serum total prostate-specific antigen (tPSA) levels was that early detection of prostate tumors would lead to timely intervention and reduced prevalence of disease.[3,4] However, screening programs have generated considerable controversy, with concerns expressed that they lead to overdiagnosis and overtreatment of prostate cancer and associated harms. The United States Preventive Services Task Force has recently issued a recommendation against screening for prostate cancer based on PSA (prostate-specific antigen).[5] However, the balance of benefits and harms of tPSA screening remains controversial.[6]

In 1999, researchers reported that the prostate cancer antigen 3 gene (PCA3; also known as DD3) was highly overexpressed in prostate cancer relative to normal prostate or benign prostatic hyperplasia tissue.[7] Subsequently, noninvasive PCA3 tests on messenger RNA (ribonucleic acid) from urine were developed.

In April 2012, a draft Comparative Effectiveness Review (CER), PCA3 Testing for the Diagnosis and Management of Prostate Cancer, was completed. The review had two aims. The first was to evaluate the comparative effectiveness of replacing or supplementing existing testing approaches for decisionmaking on when to biopsy (Key Question 1) or rebiopsy (Key Question 2) men at risk for prostate cancer. Key Questions 1 and 2 were as follows.

Key Question 1: In patients with elevated tPSA and/or an abnormal digital rectal examination (DRE) who are candidates for initial prostate biopsy, what is the comparative effectiveness of PCA3 testing as a replacement for, or supplement to, standard tests, including diagnostic accuracy (clinical validity) for prostate cancer, intermediate outcomes (e.g., improved decisionmaking about biopsy), and long-term health outcomes (clinical utility), including mortality/morbidity, quality of life, and potential harms?

Key Question 2: In patients with elevated PSA and/or an abnormal DRE who are candidates for repeat prostate biopsy (when all previous biopsies were negative), what is the comparative effectiveness of PCA3 testing as a replacement for, or supplement to, standard tests, including diagnostic accuracy (clinical validity) for prostate cancer, intermediate outcomes (e.g., improved decisionmaking about biopsy), and long-term health outcomes (clinical utility), including mortality/morbidity, quality of life, and potential harms?

The second aim of the review (Key Question 3) was to evaluate the comparative effectiveness of replacing or supplementing existing approaches for categorizing men with a positive prostate cancer biopsy as having high- or low-risk cancer and making decisions about treatment (e.g., active surveillance or aggressive therapy). Key Question 3 was as follows.

Key Question 3: In patients with a positive biopsy for prostate cancer who are being evaluated to distinguish between indolent and aggressive disease, what is the effectiveness of using PCA3 testing alone, or in combination with the standard prognostic workup (e.g., tumor volume, Gleason score, clinical staging) or monitoring tests (e.g., tPSA, PSA velocity), with regard to diagnostic accuracy (clinical validity) for aggressive (high-risk) prostate cancer, intermediate outcomes (e.g., improved decisionmaking about prognosis and triage for active surveillance and/or aggressive treatment), and long-term health outcomes (clinical utility), including mortality/morbidity, quality of life, and potential harms?

The CER analyses revealed that PCA3 had improved diagnostic accuracy compared with tPSA in identifying the presence or absence of prostate cancer, with no differences resulting from biopsy status (initial vs. repeat biopsy). However, the strength of evidence was low. The CER data from matched studies were insufficient to answer all other questions posed. In addition, issues were raised about methodological flaws in current research approaches, including risk of biases related to selection of study subjects, the generally poor quality of individual studies, and the lack of longitudinal studies to investigate the impact of early decisionmaking on long-term health outcomes.

Several important evidence gaps were identified in the draft PCA3 CER:

- Lack of information on how much improvement in diagnostic accuracy is needed for any new test to impact biopsy decisionmaking
- Lack of information on the potential of adding PCA3 alone or with other biomarkers to change decisionmaking in practice
- Lack of information on how PCA3 compares in terms of diagnostic accuracy and clinical utility with the two more frequently used add-on tests (free PSA, PSA velocity) that have appeared in guidance documents
- Need for matched studies (studies in which results of testing between PCA3 and the comparators of interest are performed and reported on the same individuals rather than only on groups of individuals) not derived from "convenience" populations (e.g., biopsy referral centers) and more data on how key demographic factors (family history, race) impact the performance of PCA3 and comparators
- Need for outcome studies to determine how well PCA3 and other comparators used to categorize risk as insignificant/indolent or aggressive predict the behavior of tumors over time
- Lack of information on a range of methodological and statistical questions related to modeling, assessing the impact of verification bias, identifying most effective cutoffs for tests based on ROC (reviewer operating characteristic) analysis, and designs for future studies

The analytical frameworks that guided the draft PCA3 CER are provided in Figures A and B.

Figure A. Future research needs for PCA3 testing: analytic framework for PCA3 as a diagnostic indicator for biopsy or rebiopsy in patients with elevated tPSA and/or abnormal digital rectal examination (Key Questions 1 and 2)

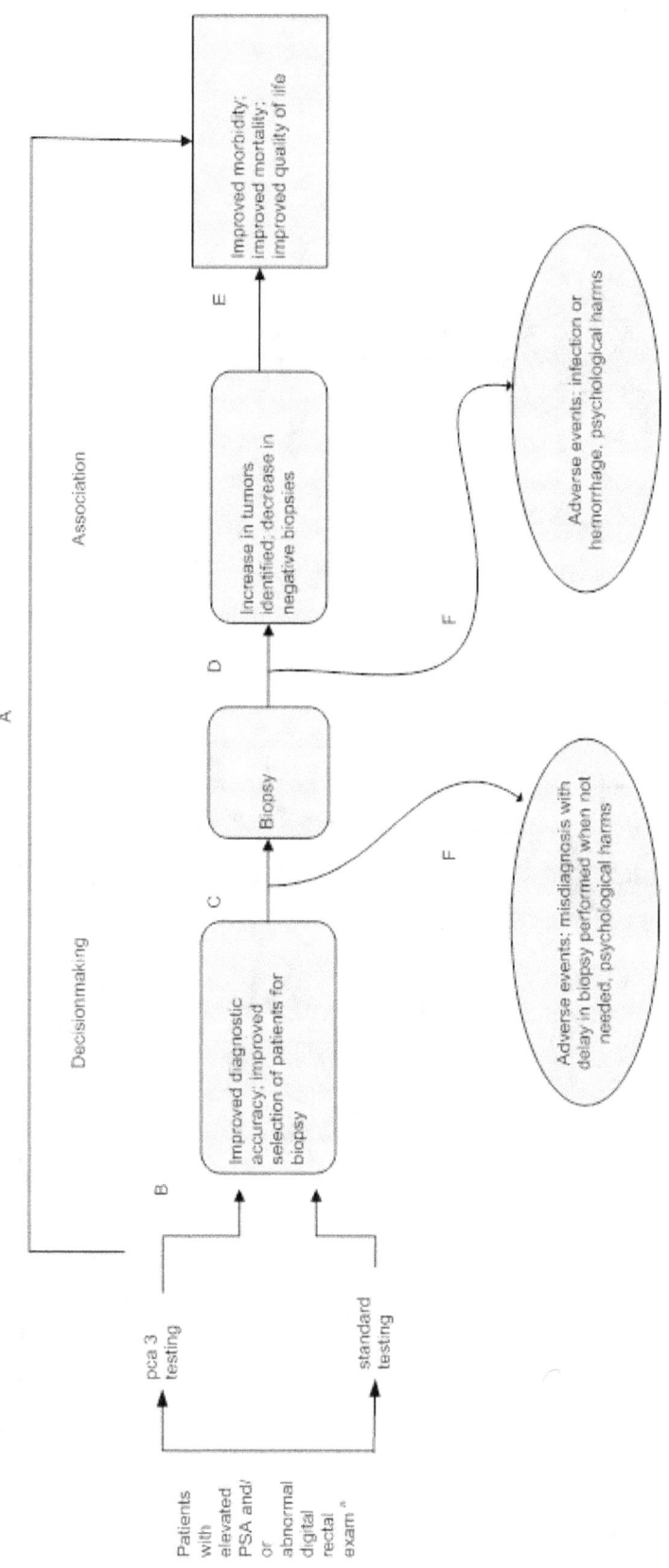

Abbreviations: PCA3 = prostate cancer antigen 3 gene; PSA = prostate-specific antigen; tPSA = total prostate-specific antigen
[a]Patients may be evaluated for initial biopsy after one or more negatives.
Note: For link B, PCA3 shows increased diagnostic accuracy compared with tPSA (low strength of evidence); for all other links (comparators and outcomes), strength of evidence is insufficient.

Figure B. Future research needs for PCA3 testing: analytic framework for PCA3 used to distinguish indolent versus aggressive prostate cancer (Key Question 3)

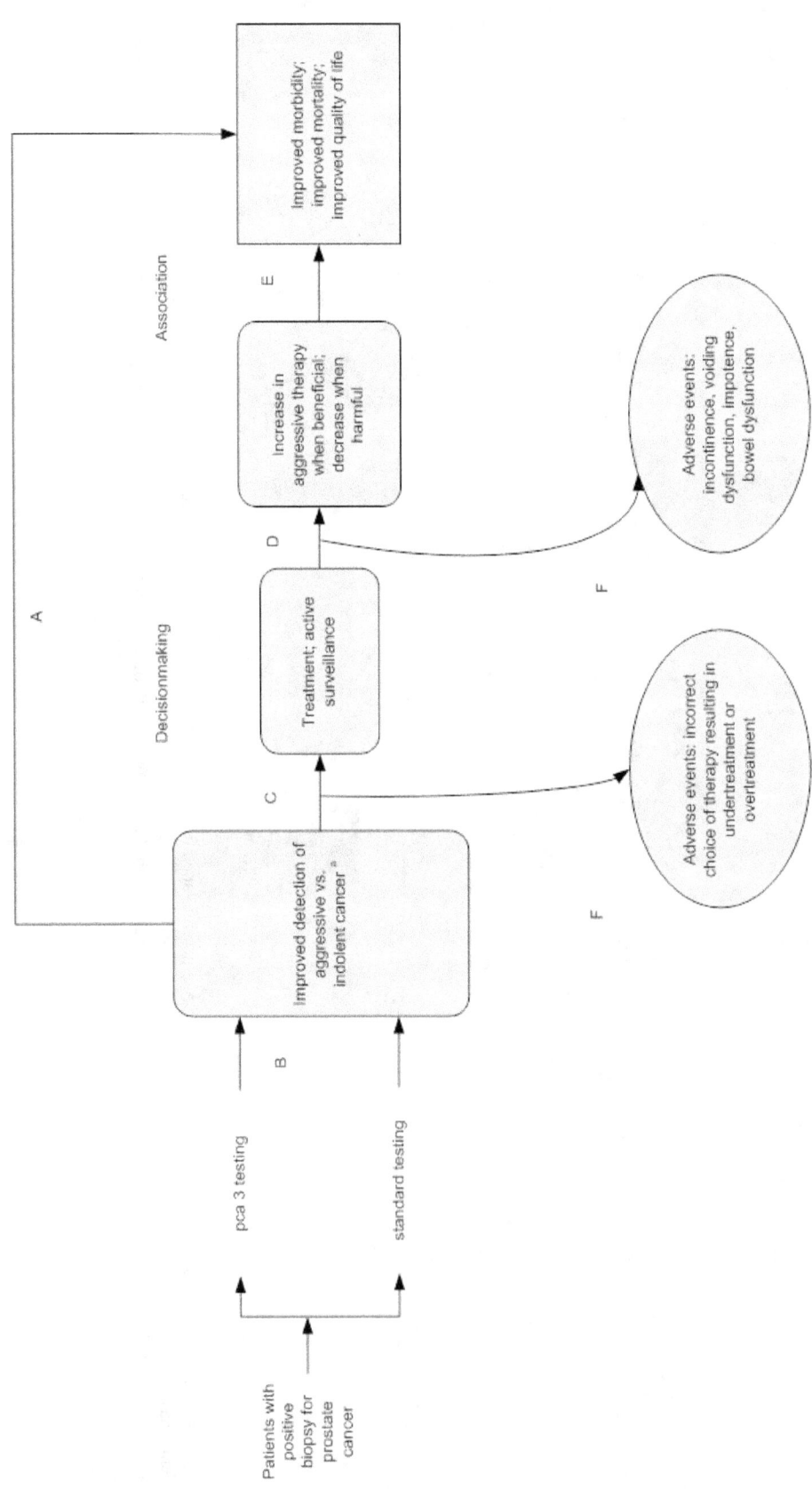

Abbreviation: PCA3 = prostate cancer antigen 3 gene
[a]Diagnostic accuracy
Note: Strength of evidence is insufficient for all links (comparators and outcomes).

Methods

Evidence gaps identified from the draft PCA3 CER, an update of the literature search, and a Stakeholder Panel were used to develop future research needs and preliminary questions. The Stakeholder Panel consisted of a group of eight individuals representing diverse perspectives, including methodological/research expertise, clinical experience (urology, oncology, epidemiology), clinical laboratory experience, and patient and payer representation. The Evidence-based Practice Center (EPC) staff compiled a list of research needs and questions, taking the Stakeholders' comments into consideration. Through an iterative process including the use of teleconferences and SurveyMonkey®, an online survey tool, the EPC staff refined the research needs, and then the Stakeholder Panel prioritized them. In selecting criteria for prioritizing research needs and research questions, the Effective Health Care (EHC) Program Selection Criteria[8] were modified to be applicable to primary research rather than to systematic reviews. The modified EHC Program Selection Criteria were distributed to the Stakeholders each time they were asked to prioritize research needs or research questions.

Research questions for each of the three research needs that were ranked the highest were generated from the CER and also through teleconferences and online input from Stakeholders. Research questions were characterized using the PICOTS (population, interventions, comparators, outcomes, timing, setting) framework.[9] The Stakeholders again used SurveyMonkey® to prioritize the research questions for each research need. The EPC, with input from the Stakeholder Panel, evaluated a variety of study designs for their potential to address the research needs and questions in accordance with the recent Future Research Needs methods report authored by the EPCs for the Agency for Healthcare Research and Quality.[10]

Results

A total of nine research needs were identified through a combination of the CER findings, updated literature search, and input from the Stakeholders. Through the online prioritization process, the EPC generated a list of the three highest priority research needs, taking all Stakeholder comments into account. The Stakeholders prioritized the list of seven research questions (four for Research Need 1, two for Research Need 2, and one for Research Need 3) within each research need, resulting in six priority research questions (three for Research Need 1, two for Research Need 2, and one for Research Need 3). EPC staff evaluated the appropriateness of various study designs to address the research needs and further prioritized the research needs. The final prioritized list of three research needs, with associated research questions and PICOTS, is presented in Table A.

Discussion

Based on the draft 2012 CER PCA3 Testing for the Diagnosis and Management of Prostate Cancer and with input from a diverse group of Stakeholders, a 10-step process was used for identifying and prioritizing clinically important research needs and research questions. The Stakeholders agreed with the findings of the CER and recognized that work needed to be done to better understand the clinical performance, impact on decisionmaking, and long-term health outcomes of PCA3 testing.

Given the complexity of topics discussed in the CER, the decision to limit the future research needs project to items within the clinical scope of testing, and to not address more general methodological and statistical issues, assured focus to the project.

Table A. Priority PCA3 research needs with research questions and PICOTS

Rank	Research Need	Preliminary Research Questions	Population	Intervention	Comparator	Outcome	Timing	Setting
1	Information on the comparative performance of PCA3 and currently used biomarkers to detect prostate cancer; "matched studies" on comparators	1. What is the comparative effectiveness of PCA3 compared with the 2 commonly used add-on tests of fPSA and tPSA velocity/doubling time in predicting prostate biopsy results?	Patients at risk for prostate cancer based on elevated PSA and/or abnormal DRE	PCA3 testing	fPSA and PSA velocity/doubling time	Positive biopsy	Any duration of followup	All settings
		2. What are PCA3's diagnostic performance characteristics in patients with elevated tPSA levels?	Patients at risk for prostate cancer based on elevated PSA and/or abnormal DRE	PCA3 testing	tPSA	Positive biopsy	Any duration of followup	All settings
		3. What is the comparative effectiveness of PCA3 compared with externally validated nomograms in predicting prostate biopsy results?	Patients at risk for prostate cancer based on elevated PSA and/or abnormal DRE	PCA3 testing	Externally validated nomograms	Positive biopsy	Any duration of followup	All settings
2	Studies on how PCA3 actually helps in biopsy or treatment decisionmaking[a]	1. What information does PCA3 provide about the aggressiveness of prostate cancer? Do positive results correlate with tumors with aggressive features on biopsy or upgrading of tumors on prostatectomy? Do negative results correlate with tumors that may not require identification or aggressive treatment?	Patients with elevated PCA3 values	PCA3 testing	Current standard of care without PCA3 testing	Features of aggressive tumor on biopsy; upgrading of tumor on prostatectomy	Any duration of followup	All settings
		2. Does the addition of PCA3, either alone or in combination with other markers, change prostate cancer biopsy or treatment decisionmaking for the patient or physician?	Patients with PCA3 values available for making decisions about biopsy or about applying active surveillance vs. aggressive therapy	PCA3 testing	Current standard of care without PCA3 testing	Decision to biopsy or wait; decision to initiate aggressive therapy or elect to be followed with active surveillance	Any duration of followup	All settings
3	Information on impact of PCA3 in biopsy decisionmaking on long-term health outcomes	1. Does the addition of PCA3 testing change long-term health outcomes in prostate screening?	Patients electing to be screened for prostate cancer using PSA and/or DRE	PCA3 testing	Current standard of care without PCA3 testing	Mortality, morbidity, quality of life	Any duration of followup	All settings

Abbreviations: DRE = digital rectal examination; fPSA = free prostate-specific antigen; PCA3 = prostate cancer antigen 3 gene; PICOTS = population, interventions, comparators, outcomes, timing, setting; PSA = prostate-specific antigen; tPSA = total prostate-specific antigen

[a]This gap includes lack of information on the correlation between PCA3 results and tumor aggressiveness, which is critical in understanding how decisions will be made.

ES-6

There were several strengths to our process. First, Stakeholder Panel members came from a wide variety of relevant disciplines, which was important to provide a balanced and broad perspective on the research needs being discussed. Second, the use of a variety of interactive communication approaches, including a one-on-one orientation to the project, two teleconferences, and emails and Internet surveys, allowed work to proceed in an efficient and timely manner. Third, the Stakeholders actively and vigorously participated in all phases of the project.

In evaluating the Stakeholders' prioritization of the research needs, a logical pattern evolved that seemed to fit well with the development and credentialing of a new diagnostic test. Highest priority went to establishing the diagnostic accuracy of the test. This is a highly pragmatic starting point, since without a clinically validated signal, risk of failure in further exploration of the use of a new test is high. Second, priority went to defining what information the test signal conveyed about the aggressiveness of missed or identified disease and how this information might be used in decisionmaking. It is likely that a test that had a weak signal or that was poor at discriminating between indolent and aggressive disease might not convince physicians or patients in either real or simulated studies to make changes in management choices. Hence, the value of such a test would obviously be limited. Finally, in order to understand how a test impacts health outcomes, there is a need for either clinical studies or a strong chain of evidence based on carefully selected and documented surrogates for predicting outcomes.

It would be difficult to perform the randomized clinical trial that would be required to establish the ultimate benefits and risks of PCA3 testing. Therefore, the Stakeholders provided the pragmatic direction of considering mechanisms for looking at chains of evidence that could provide information about long-term health outcomes without waiting for completion of a long-term clinical trial. Panel suggestions included the correlation of PCA3 testing with prognostic features on biopsy or with changes in grading between biopsy and prostatectomy, short-term clinical studies fashioned after the REDUCE (Reduction by Dutasteride of Prostate Cancer Events) trial but with PCA3 testing as an intervention, and add-on studies to ongoing investigations of active surveillance in carefully chosen patients.

Conclusions

The following three prioritized research needs and six research questions were identified.

Research Need 1: Information on the comparative performance of PCA3 and currently used biomarkers to detect prostate cancer; "matched studies" on comparators.

- **Research Question 1.1:** What is the comparative effectiveness of PCA3 compared with the two commonly used add-on tests of fPSA (free prostate-specific antigen) and tPSA velocity/doubling time in predicting prostate biopsy results?
- **Research Question 1.2:** What are PCA3's diagnostic performance characteristics in patients with elevated tPSA levels?
- **Research Question 1.3:** What is the comparative effectiveness of PCA3 compared with externally validated nomograms in predicting prostate biopsy results?

Research Need 2: Studies on how PCA3 actually helps in biopsy or treatment decisionmaking.

- **Research Question 2.1:** What information does PCA3 provide about the aggressiveness of prostate cancer? Do positive results correlate with tumors with aggressive features on biopsy or upgrading of tumors on prostatectomy? Do negative results correlate with tumors that may not require identification or aggressive treatment?

- **Research Question 2.2:** Does the addition of PCA3, either alone or in combination with other markers, change prostate cancer biopsy or treatment decisionmaking for the patient or physician?

Research Need 3: Information on impact of PCA3 in biopsy decisionmaking on long-term health outcomes.

- Research Question 3.1: Does the addition of PCA3 testing change long-term health outcomes in prostate screening?

References

1. Jemal A, Siegel R, Xu J, et al. Cancer statistics, 2010. CA Cancer J Clin. 2010 Sep-Oct;60(5):277-300. PMID: 20610543.

2. Freedland SJ. Screening, risk assessment, and the approach to therapy in patients with prostate cancer. Cancer. 2011 Mar 15;117(6):1123-35. PMID: 20960523.

3. Sutcliffe P, Hummel S, Simpson E. Use of classical and novel biomarkers as prognostic risk factors for localised prostate cancer: a systematic review. Health Technol Assess. 2009;13:1-260.

4. Tosoian J. Loeb S. PSA and beyond: the past, present, and future of investigative biomarkers for prostate cancer. Scientific World J. 2010;10:1919-31. PMID: 20890581.

5. Moyer VA. Screening for Prostate Cancer: U.S. Preventive Services Task Force Recommendation Statement. Ann Intern Med. 2012 May 21 [Epub ahead of print]. PMID: 22615453.

6. Draisma G, Boer R, Otto SJ, et al. Lead times and overdetection due to prostate-specific antigen screening: estimates from the European Randomized Study of Screening for Prostate Cancer. J Natl Cancer Inst. 2003;95(12):868-78.

7. Bussmakers MJ, van Bokhoven A, Verhaegh GW, et al. DD3: a new prostate-specific gene, highly overexpressed in prostate cancer. Cancer Res. 1999 Dec 1;59(23):5975-9.

8. Whitlock EP, Lopez SA, Chang S, et al. AHRQ Series Paper 3: Identifying, selecting, and refining topics for comparative effectiveness systematic reviews: AHRQ and the Effective Health-Care program. J Clin Epidemiol. 2010;63:491-501.

9. Robinson KA, Saldanha IJ, Mckoy NA. Frameworks for Determining Research Gaps During Systematic Reviews. Methods Future Research Needs Report No. 2. (Prepared by the Johns Hopkins University Evidence-based Practice Center under Contract No. HHSA 290-2007-10061-I.) AHRQ Publication No. 11-EHC043-EF. Rockville, MD: Agency for Healthcare Research and Quality. June 2011. www.effectivehealthcare.ahrq.gov/reports/final.cfm.

10. Carey T, Sanders G, Viswanathan M, et al. Framework for Considering Study Designs for Future Research Needs. Methods Future Research Needs Paper No. 8. (Prepared by the RTI–UNC Evidence-based Practice Center under Contract No. 290-2007-10056-I.) AHRQ Publication No. 12-EHC048-EF. Rockville, MD: Agency for Healthcare Research and Quality. March 2012. www.effectivehealthcare.ahrq.gov/reports/final.cfm.

Background

Clinical Context

Cancer of the prostate is the second most common cancer and the second leading cause of cancer deaths in men in the United States.[1] Most patients have indolent tumors, and may live for years with no or minimal effects, ultimately dying of other causes.[2] The lifetime risk of being diagnosed with prostate cancer is 16 percent, but the lifetime risk of dying from the disease is only three percent.[3] However, some patients have aggressive tumors that spread beyond the prostate, resulting in significant morbidity and death.

The rationale for prostate cancer screening using serum total prostate specific antigen (tPSA) levels[4,5] was that early detection of prostate tumors would lead to timely intervention and reduced prevalence of disease. However, screening programs have generated considerable controversy, with concerns expressed that they lead to over-diagnosis and over-treatment of prostate cancer and associated harms.[2] The United States Preventive Services Task Force has recently issued a recommendation against PSA-based screening for prostate cancer;[6] however, the balance of benefits and harms of tPSA screening remains controversial.[7]

In 1999, researchers reported that the prostate cancer antigen 3 gene (*PCA3*; also known as *DD3*), was highly overexpressed in prostate cancer relative to normal prostate or benign prostatic hyperplasia tissue.[8] Subsequently, noninvasive PCA3 tests on messenger RNA from urine were developed. Two proposed intended uses of PCA3 and comparator tests were to inform decisionmaking about biopsy or rebiopsy of men with elevated tPSA and/or other risk factors. A third purpose was to inform decisions about treatment (e.g., active surveillance, prostatectomy, radiotherapy) by classifying disease in men with positive biopsies as low risk (indolent) or high risk (aggressive). The U.S. Food and Drug Administration recently approved a PCA3 assay for use in men with one or more previous negative biopsies to inform decisionmaking about repeat biopsy.

In April 2012, a draft comparative effectiveness review (CER) on PCA3 Testing in the Diagnosis and Management of Prostate Cancer was completed. The review had two aims. The first was to evaluate the comparative effectiveness of replacing or supplementing existing testing approaches for decisionmaking on when to biopsy (KQ 1) or rebiopsy (KQ 2) men at risk for prostate cancer. Key Questions 1 and 2 were as follows:

- **KQ 1:** In patients with elevated tPSA and/or an abnormal DRE who are candidates for initial prostate biopsy, what is the comparative effectiveness of PCA3 testing as a replacement for, or supplement to, standard tests, including diagnostic accuracy (clinical validity) for prostate cancer, intermediate outcomes (e.g., improved decisionmaking about biopsy), and long-term health outcomes (clinical utility), including mortality/morbidity, quality of life, and potential harms?

- **KQ 2:** In patients with elevated PSA and/or an abnormal DRE who are candidates for repeat prostate biopsy (when all previous biopsies were negative), what is the comparative effectiveness of PCA3 testing as a replacement for, or supplement to, standard tests, including diagnostic accuracy (clinical validity) for prostate cancer, intermediate outcomes (e.g., improved decisionmaking about biopsy), and long-term health outcomes (clinical utility), including mortality/ morbidity, quality of life, and potential harms?

The second aim of the review was to evaluate the comparative effectiveness of replacing or supplementing existing approaches for categorizing prostate cancer biopsy-positive men as having high- or low-risk cancer, and making decisions about treatment (e.g., active surveillance or aggressive therapy; KQ 3). Key Question 3 was as follows:

- **KQ 3:** In patients with a positive biopsy for prostate cancer who are being evaluated to distinguish between indolent and aggressive disease, what is the effectiveness of using PCA3 testing alone, or in combination with the standard prognostic workup (e.g., tumor volume, Gleason score, clinical staging) or monitoring tests (e.g., PSA, PSA velocity), with regard to diagnostic accuracy (clinical validity) for aggressive (high risk) prostate cancer, intermediate outcomes (e.g., improved decisionmaking about prognosis and triage for active surveillance and/or aggressive treatment) and long-term health outcomes (clinical utility), including mortality/morbidity, quality of life, and potential harms?

Summary of PCA3 CER Results and Strength of Evidence

Our analyses revealed that PCA3 had improved diagnostic accuracy compared to tPSA in identifying the presence or absence of prostate cancer, with no differences resulting from biopsy status (initial versus repeat biopsy); however, the strength of evidence for this finding was low. The draft PCA3 CER data from matched studies was insufficient to answer all other questions posed. In addition, issues were raised about methodological flaws in current research approaches, including risk of biases related to selection of study subjects, the generally poor quality of individual studies, and the lack of longitudinal studies to investigate the impact of early decisionmaking on long-term health outcomes. Evidence gaps were identified and preliminary research questions to address those gaps were posed. Conclusions by Key Question and strength of evidence are detailed in Appendix A.

PCA3 CER Evidence Gaps

There were several important evidence gaps identified in the draft PCA3 CER:

- How much improvement in diagnostic accuracy is needed for any new test to impact biopsy decisionmaking.
- The potential of adding PCA3 alone or with other biomarkers to change decisionmaking in practice.
- How PCA3 compares in terms of diagnostic accuracy and clinical utility to the two more frequently used add on tests (free PSA, PSA velocity) that have appeared in guidance documents.
- The need for matched studies (studies which in which results of testing between PCA3 and the comparators of interest are performed and reported in the same individuals rather than only in groups of individuals) not derived from "convenience" populations (e.g., biopsy referral centers), and more data on how key demographic factors (family history, race) impact on the performance of PCA3 and comparators.
- The need for outcome studies to determine how well PCA3 and other comparators used to categorize risk as insignificant/indolent or aggressive to predict the behavior of tumors over time.
- A range of methodological and statistical questions relating to modeling, assessing impact of verification bias, identifying most effective cutoffs for tests based on ROC analysis, and designs for future studies.

The analytical frameworks that guided the draft PCA3 CER are provided in Figure 1 and Figure 2.

Figure 1. Future research needs for PCA3 testing: analytic framework for PCA3 as a diagnostic indicator for biopsy or re-biopsy in patients with elevated tPSA and/or abnormal digital rectal examination (KQ 1 and 2)

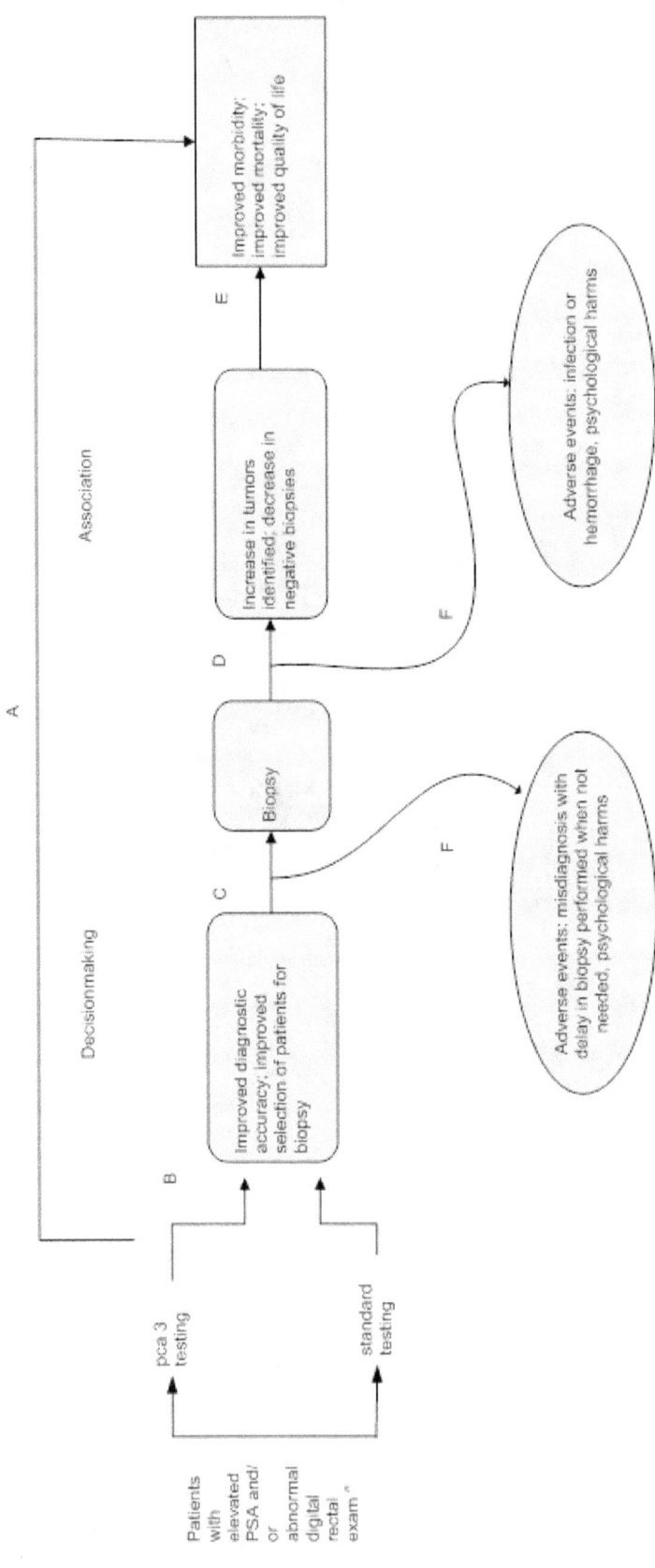

Abbreviations: PCA3 = prostate cancer antigen 3 gene; PSA = prostate-specific antigen; tPSA = total prostate-specific antigen
[a]Patients may be evaluated for initial biopsy or rebiopsy after one or more negatives.
Note: For link B, PCA3 shows increased diagnostic accuracy compared to tPSA (low strength of evidence); for all other links (comparators and outcomes) strength of evidence is insufficient.

Figure 2. Future research needs for PCA3 testing: analytic framework for PCA3 used to distinguish indolent versus aggressive prostate cancer (KQ3)

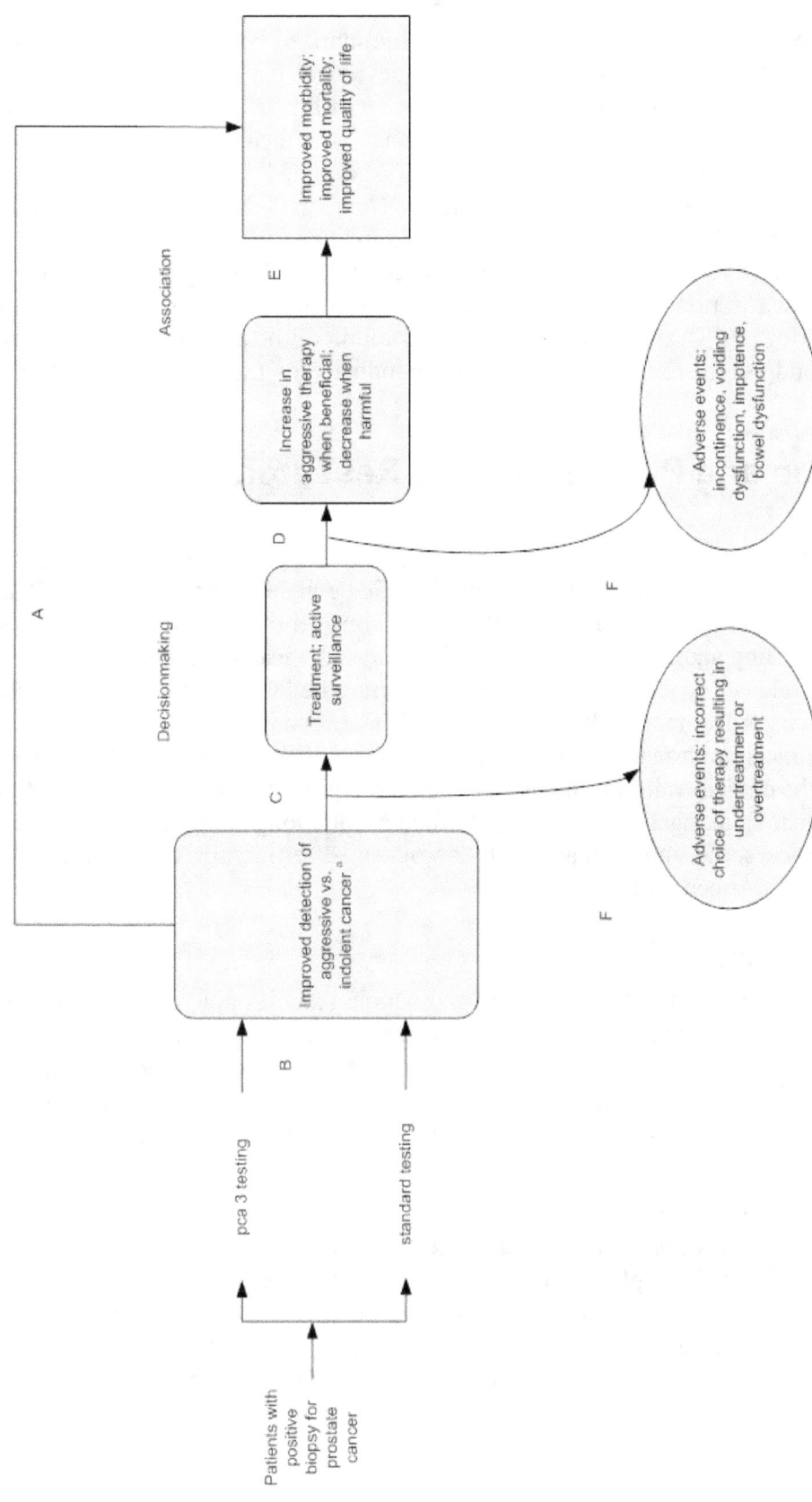

Abbreviation: PCA3 = prostate cancer antigen 3 gene
[a]Diagnostic accuracy
Note: Strength of evidence insufficient for all links (comparators and outcomes).

Methods

Figure 3 outlines the steps of the process, briefly summarized here, which was used to conduct the PCA3 future research needs project. First, evidence gaps identified from the draft CER on PCA3 Testing in the Diagnosis and Management of Prostate Cancer were used to develop future research needs and preliminary questions. After the draft CER was completed, the literature search was updated and ClinicalTrials.gov was searched to identify any ongoing research studies that might address the research needs. Next, an eight-member Stakeholder Panel was convened, comprised of individuals with expertise and experience relevant to the topic under review. Stakeholders were charged with prioritizing research needs and generating and prioritizing research questions. Research needs and research questions were prioritized online using the SurveyMonkey® Web site. Finally, the exploration of the appropriateness of various study designs to address the research questions was conducted by the EPC. Details of these steps follow.

Identification and Prioritization of Research Needs

Project Scope

The PCA3 CER project team collaboratively identified evidence gaps for the draft CER. Two types of research needs were identified from these gaps: one set that focused on clinical issues specific to PCA3 testing and a second set that focused on statistical and methodological issues and were broadly relevant to the study of new biomarkers. The PCA3 Future Research Needs (FRN) team, with input from the AHRQ Task Order Officer, made the decision to focus on the issues of direct clinical importance in understanding the use of PCA3 testing. These included issues related to the clinical validity (diagnostic accuracy) of the test, as well as to its clinical utility (use in decisionmaking and impact on intermediate and long-term health outcomes). For informational purposes, the statistical and methodological issues identified in the draft PCA3 CER are presented in Appendix B.

Literature Search Update

To identify any recent, important published and ongoing studies potentially addressing the PCA3 research needs, a literature search was conducted on May 15, 2012, using MEDLINE® (via PubMed®), Embase.com, the Cochrane Library, and the ClinicalTrials.gov databases, as well as the American Society of Clinical Oncology conference abstracts. The search strategy captured studies published since August 1, 2011, and is provided in Appendix C.

Criteria for Prioritization

In developing criteria for prioritization, the Effective Health Care (EHC) Program Selection Criteria[9] were modified to be applicable to primary research, rather than to systematic reviews of original research. They keep the spirit of the EHC criteria, but are more succinct. Table 1 provides a list of the prioritization criteria, which were used by the Stakeholder Panel when prioritizing the research needs and research questions relevant to this project.

Figure 3. Process flow diagram for PCA3 FRN project

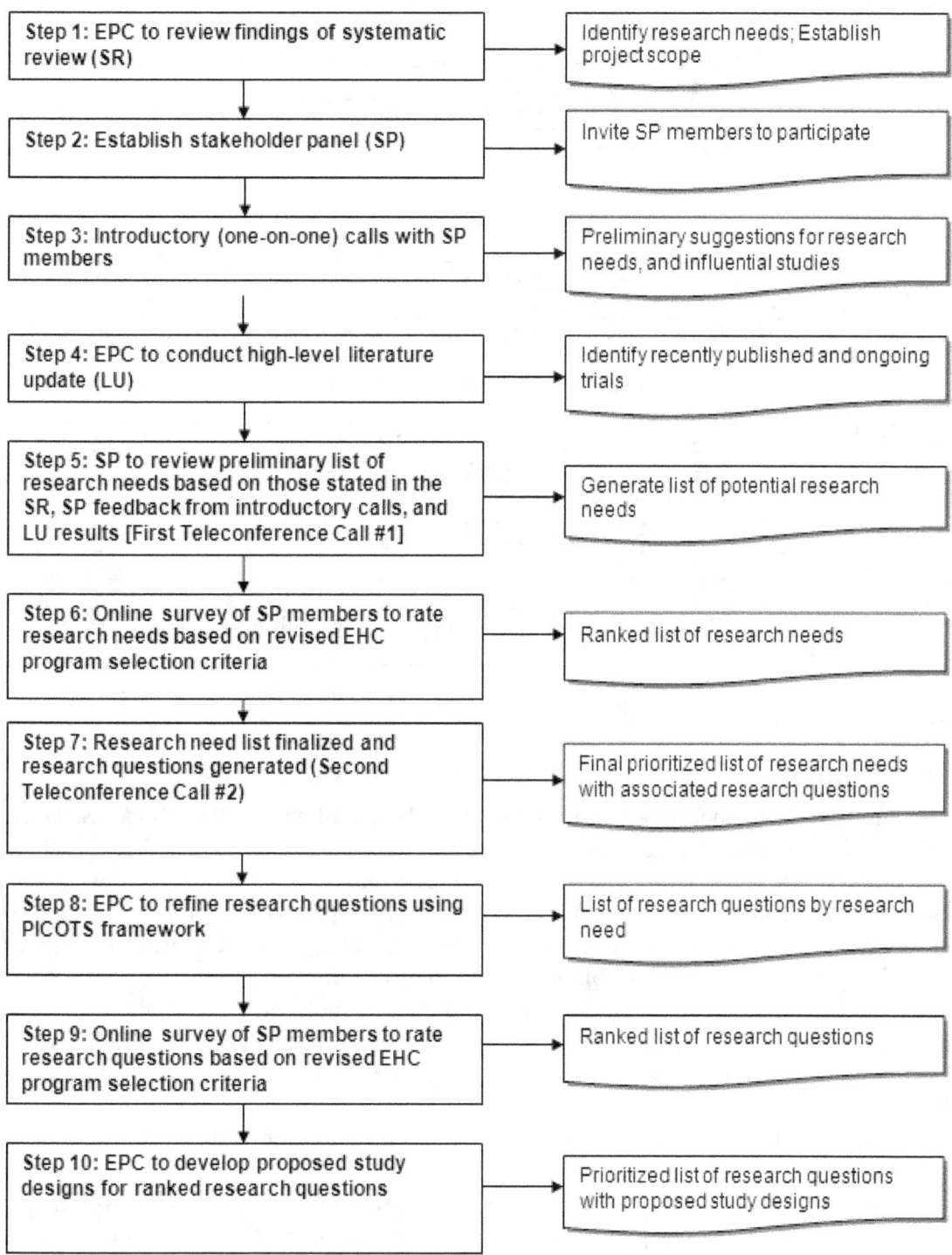

Abbreviations: EHC = effective health care; EPC = Evidence-based Practice Center

Table 1. Prioritization criteria for PCA3 research needs and proposed research studies

Category	Criterion
Current importance	• Incorporates both clinical benefits and harms.
	• Represents important variation in clinical care due to controversy/uncertainty regarding appropriate care.
	• Addresses high costs to consumers, patients, health-care systems, or payers.
	• Utility of available evidence limited by changes in practice, e.g., disease detection.

Potential for significant health impact	• Potential for significant health impact:
	    – To improve <u>health outcomes</u>.
	    – To reduce <u>significant variation</u> related to quality of care.
	    – To reduce <u>unnecessary burden</u> on those with health-care problems.

	• Potential for significant economic impact, reducing unnecessary or excessive costs.
	• Potential for evidence-based change.
	• Potential risk from inaction, i.e., lack of evidence for decisionmaking produces unintended harms
	• Addresses inequities, vulnerable populations, patient subgroups with differential impact (e.g., by age).
Incremental value	• Adds useful new information to existing portfolio of research on topic OR
	• Validates existing research when body of evidence is scant.
Feasibility	*Factors to be considered:*
	• Interest among researchers.
	• Duration.
	• Cost.
	• Methodological complexity (e.g., do existing methods need to be refined?).
	• Implementation difficulty.
	• Facilitating factors.
	• Potential funders.

Engagement of Stakeholders, Researchers, Funders

Central to the methodology of this report was the use of a multidisciplinary Stakeholder Panel to identity and prioritize research needs and research questions. The Panel included individuals interested in comparative effectiveness research and who were knowledgeable about current research on PCA3. They consisted of eight participants (including two Federal representatives) representing diverse perspectives, including methodological/research expertise, clinical experience (urology, oncology, epidemiology), clinical laboratory experience, and patient and payer representation. The Stakeholder Panel included individuals with specific experience on the identification and treatment of prostate cancer. As proscribed by AHRQ, conflict of interest forms were completed by all members of the Stakeholder Panel and staff on this project.

The Stakeholders participated in a brief (i.e., 30-minute) orientation call with the team leader, who framed the topic and requested preliminary suggestions on further research needs. In addition, Stakeholders participated in two teleconference calls (1 hour each) over the course of the project, during which they provided input, first on the research needs and then the research questions. Alternative calls were scheduled as necessary with members who were unable to participate during the panel calls. All teleconference call materials were distributed a few days prior to scheduled calls. Interim communications were carried out by email.

The main role of the Stakeholder Panel was to refine and then prioritize, using an online survey, the list of research needs generated from the CER and from feedback obtained in the orientation calls. The Stakeholders also helped to refine, and then prioritized, a list of potential research questions to address the highest priority research needs.

Methods for Ranking Research Needs and Questions

Research needs were ranked via the SurveyMonkey® Web site. The Stakeholder Panel was sent a link to the Web site where they ranked the research needs from 3, for a ranking of first, to 1, for a ranking of third. The research need with the largest number of points was assigned the highest priority. Stakeholders also had the opportunity to provide comments about the survey. The same process was used by Stakeholders to prioritize the research questions associated with each research need.

Research Question Development and Study Design Considerations

Research questions for each research need were generated based on the original CER and input from Stakeholders during the orientation call, the two followup teleconferences, and by on-line solicitation. The project team compiled a final list of research questions for the three highest priority research needs; these were then prioritized by the Stakeholders according to importance.

The research needs and research questions were characterized according to the PICOTS framework using patient population (P), intervention (I), comparison (C), outcomes (O), timing (T), and setting (S). This approach is consistent with the guidance produced by the John Hopkins University EPC on behalf of AHRQ.[10]

Study design considerations were handled by the EPC in accordance with the recent Future Research Needs methods report authored by the RTI-UNC EPC on behalf of AHRQ.[11] The following criteria were used to evaluate the appropriateness of any one study design to address a research need:

- Advantages of the study design for producing a valid result;
- Resource use, size, and duration;
- Ethical, legal, and social issues;
- Availability of data or ability to recruit

The PCA3 FRN team relied on this framework as a guide during discussions of the least biased study design that was likely to be feasible and affordable for each research question. The Stakeholder Panel provided insight into how future research agendas and proposed studies to address research needs fit within these prespecified criteria.

Results

Literature Search Update

The literature search update captured 107 studies published since August 1, 2011. A table of primary studies, new abstracts, and ongoing clinical trials deemed relevant to the research needs and research questions is provided in Appendix D.

Research Needs

The orientation calls to each member of the Stakeholder Panel were conducted between May 14 and 18, 2012. The first teleconference with all the Stakeholders occurred in two sessions: the first with four Stakeholders participating on May 21, 2012, and the second with six Stakeholders participating on May 29, 2012. Two Stakeholders participated in both calls. A total of nine research needs (see Appendix E) were identified through a combination of the CER findings and input from the Stakeholder panel. During the first teleconference, the Stakeholders reviewed the preliminary list of nine research needs, made the suggestion that they be more detailed rather than generic, and also discussed possible future research questions and study designs.

After the first teleconference, the Stakeholders completed the online SurveyMonkey®, ranking their top three research needs from the list of nine, using the revised EHC program selection criteria previously described. The response rate was 100 percent (n=8). Total scores ranged from 11 to 3, with a single item receiving no votes and a score of 0. The results of the first survey are provided in Appendix F.

A second teleconference was held on June 14, 2012, to discuss the results of the Stakeholders' prioritization of the research needs and to solicit input on research questions. Again, to accommodate the busy schedules of participants, calls were made at two separate times, with four Stakeholders participating in a morning session and three in an afternoon session (a total of 6 of 8 Stakeholders participated; the remaining two provided followup input in one-on-one calls with the team leader).

Based on an evaluation of scores, there was no single, clear cut-off point on which to distinguish high- from low-priority items. In the teleconference discussion, the Stakeholder Panel used an empirical approach to establish this cut-off, based on the observation that a logical progression for a diagnostic assay like PCA3 was to move from an understanding of the clinical validity of the signal to informed applications of its use in decisionmaking followed by either a chain of evidence or direct evidence suggesting a positive impact on long-term health outcomes.

The top-ranked research needs were as follows:

- **Research Need 1**: Lack of information on the comparative performance of PCA3 and currently used biomarkers to detect prostate cancer; lack of "matched studies" on comparisons;
- **Research Need 8**: Lack of studies on how PCA3 actually helps in treatment decisionmaking;
- **Research Need 5**: Lack of information on the impact of PCA3 on short-term outcomes, such as biopsy decisionmaking; and
- **Research need 6**: Uncertainty of impact of PCA3 in biopsy decisionmaking on long-term health outcomes.

Based on their empirical approach, the Stakeholders suggested combining Research Needs 5 and 8 into one item addressing decisionmaking and including Research Need 6 as the final item determining the impact of PCA3 testing on long-term health outcomes.

The resulting three top-ranked research needs were as follows:

- **Research Need 1**: Lack of information on the comparative performance of PCA3 and currently used biomarkers to detect prostate cancer; lack of "matched studies" on comparisons;
- **Research Need 2**: Lack of studies on how PCA3 actually helps in biopsy or treatment decisionmaking; and
- **Research Need 3**: Uncertainty of the impact of PCA3 in biopsy decisionmaking on long-term health outcomes.

Research Need 1 addresses the diagnostic accuracy of PCA3 in comparison to other tests for prostate cancer. In the PCA3 CER, the most common comparison observed was between PCA3 and tPSA. A small number of articles described PCA3 compared to percent-free PSA or to nomograms; however, the information was either low in quality or insufficient to draw conclusions about the relative performance of these tests.

Research Need 2 addresses how understanding the aggressiveness of identified or missed tumors might be used in decisionmaking about whether to biopsy or defer and follow the patient over time, or used to determine whether a patient should be offered active surveillance versus aggressive therapy.

Research Need 3 addresses the critical question of whether PCA3 testing has an impact on long-term health outcomes. To the extent that PCA3 testing reduces the need for biopsy or identifies aggressive tumors that warrant treatment, the assay has the potential to increase benefits and reduce harms. The panel recognized that this research need might be difficult to address, but concluded that test accuracy alone would not necessarily equate to test effectiveness.

Research Questions

Research questions for each of the research needs were generated from the PCA3 CER and input from the Stakeholder Panel. Relevant research questions were the subject of discussion at both teleconferences as Stakeholders considered mechanisms for addressing the important research needs identified. Based on a Stakeholder suggestion, one research question was added to the original three from the CER for Research need 1, but none were added to the original two questions for Research Need 2 or the one question for Research Need 3.

Once the final list of research questions was compiled, Stakeholders again completed an online SurveyMonkey® to prioritize the research questions (see Appendix G). Because of the well-established hierarchal approach provided by the Stakeholders, the prioritization of research questions was modified to rate questions within each research need, rather than to generically evaluate these questions collectively across the research needs.

For Research Need 1, there were a total of four research questions, and each Stakeholder ranked the top three of most importance. For Research Need 2, the Stakeholders ranked the two questions in order of perceived importance. Research Need 3 had only one research question and was, therefore, not included for prioritization. The prioritization results for the research questions for Research Needs 1 and 2 are presented in Appendix H.

For Research Need 1, the three highest priority research questions were as follows:

- **Research Question 1.2**: What is the comparative effectiveness of PCA3 compared to the two commonly used add-on tests of fPSA and tPSA velocity/doubling time in predicting prostate biopsy results?
- **Research Question 1.1**: What are PCA3's diagnostic performance characteristics in patients with elevated tPSA levels?
- **Research Question 1.3**: What is the comparative effectiveness of PCA3 compared to externally validated nomograms in predicting prostate biopsy results?

For Research Need 2, both research questions were ranked equally, and therefore remained in the following order:

- **Research Question 2.1**: What information does PCA3 provide about the aggressiveness of prostate cancer? Do positive results correlate to tumors with aggressive features on biopsy or upgrading of tumors on prostatectomy? Do negative results correlate to tumors that may not require identification or aggressive treatment?
- **Research Question 2.2**: Does the addition of PCA3, either alone, or in combination with other markers, change prostate cancer biopsy or treatment decisionmaking for the patient or physician?

The final three research needs, in priority order, along with the associated prioritized research questions and PICOTS are presented in Table 2.

Table 2. Priority PCA3 research needs with research questions and PICOTS

Rank	Research Need	Preliminary Research Questions	Population	Intervention	Comparator	Outcome	Timing	Setting
1	Lack of information on the comparative performance of PCA3 and currently used biomarkers to detect prostate cancer; lack of "matched studies" on comparators	1. What is the comparative effectiveness of PCA3 compared to the two commonly used add-on tests of fPSA and tPSA velocity/doubling time in predicting prostate biopsy results?	Patients at risk for prostate cancer based on elevated PSA and/or abnormal DRE	PCA3 testing	fPSA and PSA velocity/doubling time	Positive biopsy	Any duration of followup will be evaluated.	All settings
		2. What are PCA3's diagnostic performance characteristics in patients with elevated tPSA levels?	Patients at risk for prostate cancer based on elevated PSA and/or abnormal DRE	PCA3 testing	tPSA	Positive biopsy	Any duration of followup will be evaluated	All settings
		3. What is the comparative effectiveness of PCA3 compared to externally validated nomograms in predicting prostate biopsy results?	Patients at risk for prostate cancer based on elevated PSA and/or abnormal DRE	PCA3 testing	Externally validated nomograms	Positive biopsy	Any duration of followup will be evaluated	All settings
2	Lack of studies on how PCA3 actually helps in biopsy or treatment decisionmaking[a]	1. What information does PCA3 provide about the aggressiveness of prostate cancer? In other words, do positive results correlate to tumors with aggressive features on biopsy or upgrading of tumors on prostatectomy? Do negative results correlate to tumors that may not require identification or aggressive treatment?	Patients with elevated PCA3 values	PCA3 testing	Current standard of care without PCA3 testing	Features of aggressive tumor on biopsy; upgrading of tumor on prostatectomy	Any duration of followup will be evaluated	All settings
		2. Does the addition of PCA3, either alone, or in combination with other markers, change prostate cancer biopsy or treatment decisionmaking for the patient or physician?	Patients with PCA3 values available for making decisions about biopsy or decision to apply active surveillance versus aggressive therapy	PCA3 testing	Current standard of care without PCA3 testing	Decision to biopsy or wait; decision to initiate aggressive therapy or to elect to be followed with active surveillance	Any duration of followup will be evaluated	All settings
3	Uncertainty of impact of PCA3 in biopsy decisionmaking on long-term health outcomes	1. Does addition of PCA3 testing change long-term health outcomes in prostate screening?	Patients electing to be screened for prostate cancer using PSA and/or digital rectal exam	PCA3 testing	Current standard of care without PCA3 testing	Mortality, morbidity, quality of life	Any duration of followup will be evaluated	All settings

Abbreviations: DRE = digital rectal examination; fPSA = free prostate-specific antigen; PCA3 = prostate cancer antigen 3 gene; PICOTS = population, interventions, comparators, outcomes, timing, setting; PSA = prostate-specific antigen; tPSA = total prostate-specific antigen

[a]This gap includes lack of information on the correlation between PCA3 results and tumor aggressiveness, which is critical in understanding how decisions will be made.

Study Designs

The PCA3 FRN team considered and evaluated a number of study designs to address the priority research needs and their associated research questions.

For the assessment of study designs for Research Need 1, the appropriateness of using diagnostic accuracy,[12,13] prospective - retrospective studies using archived samples,[14] and case control studies[15,16] to assess diagnostic performance of PCA3 were evaluated.

For the assessment of the impact of PCA3 testing on decisionmaking (Research Need 2), the study designs proposed differed for the two research questions. For Research Question 2.1, which focuses on tumor aggressiveness, rather than just the detection of tumors alone, the study designs were the same as those described for Research Need 1, Research Questions 1.1-1.3.

Research Question 2.2 addresses the issue of whether the magnitude of changes in prediction for biopsy outcomes provided by PCA3 impacts clinical decisionmaking. In this case, three kinds of studies of physician/patient response to test results were evaluated: randomized clinical trial, prospective cohort study, and physician/patient survey.

For the assessment of the impact of PCA3 testing on long-term health outcomes (Research Need 3), the appropriateness of the randomized clinical trial, prospective cohort study, and modeling were evaluated.

The specific research designs to address each research need and research question are described below and are included in Tables 3 through 6.

Study Design Evaluation

Research Need 1: Lack of information on the comparative performance of PCA3 and currently used biomarkers to detect prostate cancer; lack of "matched studies" on comparators.

- **Research Question 1.1**: What is the comparative effectiveness of PCA3 compared to the two commonly used add-on tests of fPSA and tPSA velocity/doubling time in predicting prostate biopsy results?
- **Research Question 1.2**: What are PCA3's diagnostic performance characteristics in patients with elevated tPSA levels?
- **Research Question 1.3**: What is the comparative effectiveness of PCA3 compared to externally validated nomograms in predicting prostate biopsy results?

Table 3 provides the study design evaluations for Research Questions 1.1–1.3, which were combined because they require the same basic approach. In each, the objective is to determine the comparative performance of PCA3 against the current standard of care by establishing diagnostic accuracy for each test of interest.

An ideal study to establish diagnostic accuracy would be to identify a large cohort of men being screened for prostate cancer (most commonly based on elevated PSA and/or abnormal DRE). All positive patients would be tested for analytes of interest: tPSA (repeated to assess regression to the mean), free PSA, PSA velocity, nomograms etc. All men would undergo biopsy to allow for a head to head comparison of PCA3 to currently used tests. Although it is unlikely everyone would be biopsied, as many as possible should be biopsied and reasons for dropout carefully described. It is important to note that this information was uniformly absent from studies of PCA3.

This ideal study, like most studies in the current literature, should be of matched design (comparative biomarkers are measured in the same individuals in the same setting allowing

Table 3. Study design evaluations for PCA3 Research Need 1, Research Questions 1.1–1.3

Study Design Considerations	Diagnostic Accuracy Study	Prospective-Retrospective Study	Case Control Study
Description of design	PCA3 compared to currently used tests (tPSA, free PSA, PSA velocity, externally validated nomograms without PCA3; externally validated nomograms including PCA3); clinical performance (sensitivity, specificity, positive and negative predictive values) assessed and reported in matched comparisons to a biopsy gold standard. Results of PCA3 are blinded and not used in decisionmaking.	PCA3 measured in archived samples from patients identified as biopsy-positive or biopsy-negative in a population resembling the intended use population. Not possible because of lack of urine specimen banks, but as noted in the Future Research Needs for Comparative Effectiveness of Treatments of Localized Prostate Cancer,[17] such banks are needed.	Samples from patients predefined as positive or negative for cancer are selected; testing is performed in these samples.
Advantages of study design for producing a valid result	Studies are usually cross-sectional or involve short-term followup only. Data to support this type of study may already exist, but have been incompletely analyzed and reported.	Uses available resources and data, but care must be taken to avoid incorrect handling of samples and incomplete data.	Allows use of convenience samples; results may not mimic real world use, and estimates of both sensitivity and specificity must be interpreted with extreme care.
Resource use, size, and duration	Study requires patient recruitment and informed consent with samples collected with active intervention (attentive digital rectal exam), special processing and then testing using PCA3 and correlation of results with standard testing against a biopsy gold standard. Followup or further diagnostic evaluation is not usually required. Currently, no good models exist for addressing verification bias and, therefore, data interpretation may be challenging.	Less resource-intensive and shorter than a randomized clinical trial. There may be costs associated with obtaining and using samples and data.	Less resource intense than a diagnostic accuracy study or a well performed retrospective study using repository samples reflecting the intended use population.
Ethical, legal and social issues	Minimal; the test is approved for use by FDA, for repeat biopsies. The test is not currently a practice of care standard, and so blinding should pose no dilemma.	Minimal; studies must be performed with attention to patient confidentiality and privacy.	Minimal; studies must be performed with attention to patient confidentiality and privacy.
Availability of data or ability to recruit	This is a high volume test process and burden of disease is high. Recruitment of subjects should not be difficult although future studies should learn from the comparative effectiveness review and pay more attention to the quality of data being collected.	This is currently very problematic in that urine repositories for patients subject to prostate cancer are not available.	This is currently problematic in that urine repositories for patients subject to prostate cancer are not available.

Abbreviations: FDA = U.S. Food and Drug Administration; PCA3 = prostate cancer antigen 3 gene; PSA = prostate-specific antigen; tPSA = total prostate-specific antigen
Note:
1.1 What is the comparative effectiveness of PCA3 compared to the two commonly used add-on tests of fPSA and tPSA velocity/doubling time in predicting prostate biopsy results?
1.2 What are PCA3's diagnostic performance characteristics in patients with elevated tPSA levels?
1.3 What is the comparative effectiveness of PCA3 compared to externally validated nomograms in predicting prostate biopsy results?

15

each individual to be a self-control). The data should be subject to matched analyses (e.g., McNemers test), stratified by biopsy-positive and biopsy-negative subgroups. Although all of the studies in this CER were matched, none of them were subject to a matched analysis.

It is important to note that although matched analysis is missing from the current literature on PCA3, most studies were performed using a matched design. It might be possible for individual investigators or groups of investigators to re-analyze existing data to better understand test performance. To the extent current reports have information on biopsy yield and reasons for drop-out, the ideal study may be approximated using existing data

While prospective-retrospective studies can sometimes be used to establish performance of a test using banked samples in patients with well-established demographic and clinical information, this is not possible for PCA3 testing at this time. While there are a number of biobanks of blood from patients studied for prostate cancer, no similar banks of stored urine are known to exist. Case control studies allow for testing in patients with established disease and in controls without disease. While this approach has the advantage that it often facilitates identification of samples for study, this design does not provide testing in the intended-use population, has a high risk of bias, and is generally reserved for exploratory studies only.

Research Need 2: Lack of studies on how PCA3 actually helps in biopsy or treatment decisionmaking.

- **Research Question 2.1:** What information does PCA3 provide about the aggressiveness of prostate cancer? In other words, do positive results correlate to tumors with aggressive features on biopsy or upgrading of tumors on prostatectomy? Do negative results correlate to tumors that may not require identification or aggressive treatment?

Table 4 provides the study design evaluation for Research Question 2.1 which, like the four research questions for Research Need 1, focuses on establishing the diagnostic accuracy of the PCA3 test. However, this question differs from the first three research questions by having as its endpoint the detection of indolent versus aggressive disease. Ideally, aggressiveness would be carefully defined, either using standard techniques established for biopsy (i.e., the Epstein criteria) or using information obtained by comparing biopsy results with staging results in men undergoing radical prostatectomy. Again a predefined cutoff would be selected, and test performance for predicting indolent or aggressive disease described in terms of diagnostic performance of clinical sensitivity, specificity, and predictive value of positive and negative results.

- **Research Question 2.2:** Does the addition of PCA3, either alone or in combination with other markers, change prostate cancer biopsy or treatment decisionmaking for the patient or physician?

Table 5 provides the study design evaluation for Research Question 2.2, which addresses the issue of whether the magnitude of changes in prediction for biopsy outcomes provided by PCA3 are significant enough to cause physicians or patients to make changes in either biopsy or treatment decisions. The goal of the research question would be to determine if the trade-off between reduction in biopsies and missed cancers could be communicated to physicians or patients in a manner that would allow for more informed decisions and improved outcomes.

Table 4. Study design evaluations for PCA3 Research Need 2, Research Question 2.1: What information does PCA3 provide about the aggressiveness of prostate cancer?

Study Design Considerations	Diagnostic Accuracy Study	Prospective-Retrospective Study	Case Control Study
Description of design	PCA3 compared to currently used tests (tPSA, free PSA, PSA velocity, externally validated nomograms without PCA3; externally validated nomograms including PCA3); clinical performance (sensitivity, specificity, positive and negative predictive values) assessed and reported in matched comparisons to a biopsy gold standard including information characterizing tumor aggressiveness. This can be based on biopsy findings that suggest aggressive versus indolent tumor behavior, such as the Epstein criteria, or can be based on changes in grading in patients with positive biopsy who go on to be treated by prostatectomy. Results of PCA3 are blinded and not used in decisionmaking.	PCA3 measured in archived samples from patients identified as biopsy-positive or biopsy-negative in a population resembling the intended use population. Not possible because of lack of urine specimen banks, but as noted in Future Research Needs for Comparative Effectiveness of Treatments of Localized Prostate Cancer[17] such banks are needed.	Patients predefined as positive or negative for cancer with measures of aggressiveness characterized are selected; testing is performed in these samples.
Advantages of study design for producing a valid result	Although information collected is similar to that for questions 1.1–1.3, more detailed information on results are sought allowing for information on whether identified/missed tumors are clinically significant or not.	Uses available resources and data, but care must be taken to avoid incorrect handling of samples and incomplete data.	Allows use of convenience samples; results may not mimic real world use, and estimates of both sensitivity and specificity must be interpreted with extreme care.
Resource use, size, and duration	Study requires patient recruitment and informed consent with samples collected with active intervention (attentive digital rectal exam), special processing and then testing using PCA3 and correlation of results with standard testing against a biopsy gold standard. Followup or further diagnostic evaluation is not required and so study efforts and costs are least burdensome.	Less resource-intense and shorter than a randomized clinical trial. There may be costs associated with obtaining and using samples and data.	Less resource-intense and shorter than a prospective study or a well-performed retrospective study using repository samples reflecting the intended use population.
Ethical, legal and social issues	Minimal; the test is approved for use by FDA, but is not currently a practice of care standard and so blinding should pose no dilemma.	Minimal; studies must be performed with attention to patient confidentiality and privacy.	Minimal; studies must be performed with attention to patient confidentiality and privacy.
Availability of data or ability	This is a high volume test process and burden of disease is high (although its impact controversial). Recruitment of subjects should not be difficult although future studies should learn from the comparative effectiveness review and pay more attention to the quality of data being collected.	This is currently very problematic in that urine repositories for patients subject to prostate cancer are not available.	This is currently problematic in that urine repositories for patients subject to prostate cancer are not available.

Abbreviations: FDA = U.S. Food and Drug Administration; PCA3 = prostate cancer antigen 3 gene; PSA = prostate-specific antigen; tPSA = total prostate-specific antigen

17

Table 5. Study design evaluations for PCA3 Research Need 1, Research Question 2.2: Does the addition of PCA3, either alone or in combination with other markers, change prostate cancer biopsy or treatment decisionmaking for the patient or physician?

Study Design Considerations	Randomized Clinical Trials	Prospective Cohort Study	Physician/Patient Survey
Description of design	Patients at risk for prostate cancer (initial or repeat biopsy) based on elevated tPSA and/or abnormal DRE or with positive biopsies are randomized to receive PCA3 in addition to standard testing or standard testing alone. Biopsies performed versus deferred and the yield of positive and negative results in the two arms are compared, and evidence of patients with aggressive versus indolent disease in the two arms is also compared. Features of aggressiveness can be enhanced by including studies that use standardized criteria linking results to clinical outcomes using published or unpublished, but public, information as available. In order to assess impact on patients choosing active surveillance versus aggressive therapy, experiments could be designed to add PCA3 to on-going studies of active surveillance. In addition, different PCA3 values could be compared to grading changes between biopsy and prostatectomy.	Patients with and without prostate cancer identified in an intended use population and tracked according to PCA3 status --tested or not tested, positive or negative test results). Patients followed prospectively to determine choices about biopsy and treatment.	Hypothetical scenarios for test use can be developed and evaluated in physicians or patients to determine how they might use information in comparison to current standard of care. To develop a meaningful survey, it is necessary to have good information on test performance and to consider how decision aids might be used to maximize use of testing information provided in such a survey.
Advantages of study design for producing a valid result	With proper inclusion and exclusion criteria and careful recording of results, this should provide a clear indication of how results will be used in decisionmaking and will also provide information on the outcomes of testing—how many cancers identified and what type (indolent or aggressive).	Baseline characteristics can be measured, but may not be balanced. Statistical techniques may be able to partially control potential bias.	There is a growing interest in the use of conjoint analysis to determine how medical information is used to affect management choices. Although the approach is new, it appears able to provide valuable information toward understanding how information might be used.
Resource use, size, and duration	This is likely to be a resource-intense process. Since the study is focused only on immediate decisionmaking and biopsy results, long -term followup would be interesting, but not essential, to answer the questions raised.	Resource use, size, and duration are likely to be similar to that of a randomized clinical trial.	Less resource intensive and shorter than a prospective study.
Ethical, legal and social issues	Minimal; although the test has been approved by FDA for repeat biopsy (previous negative biopsy patients), there is no information on health care outcomes, hence the need for study.	Minimal; although the test has been approved by FDA for repeat biopsy (previous negative biopsy patients), there is no information on health care outcomes, hence the need for study.	None. This type of survey presents no ethical, legal, or social issues.
Availability of data or ability to recruit	Biopsy or treatment choice is commonly encountered in urological practice; the area is one of considerable physician and patient interest; recruitment would be expected to be relatively straightforward.	Biopsy or treatment choice is commonly encountered in urological practice; the area is one of considerable physician and patient interest; recruitment would be expected to be relatively straight forward.	This is an area of considerable interest to both physicians and patients; recruitment should be relatively straightforward.

Abbreviations: DRE = digital rectal examination FDA = U.S. Food and Drug Administration; PCA3 = prostate cancer antigen 3 gene; PSA = prostate-specific antigen; tPSA = total prostate-specific antigen

While an optimal manner of looking at this issue would be by performing a randomized clinical trial looking at management decisions with and without use of PCA3, alternative techniques might be to perform a prospective cohort study or to use surveys or conjoint analysis to approximate decisionmaking in the face of varying test performance. Surveys or conjoint analyses are predicated on having good data about the comparative performance of the prognostic tools currently available, and would only be as reliable as performance estimates derived from data provided to answer research questions 1.1–1.3 and 2.1.

Research Need 3: Uncertainty of impact of PCA3 in biopsy decisionmaking on long-term health outcomes.

Research Question 3.1: Does addition of PCA3 testing change long-term health outcomes in prostate screening?

Table 6 provides the study design evaluations for Research Question 3.1, which focuses on the bottom line: Does PCA3 testing change long-term health outcomes? The gold standard for making this determination would be to perform a randomized controlled clinical trial, comparing management of patients with and without PCA3 and following a large number of patients over long periods of time to determine actual impact of testing on morbidity, mortality, and quality of life. An alternative would be a prospective cohort study. Stakeholders recognized the challenges such studies would present; however, as one Stakeholder noted, *accuracy* of testing does not assure *effectiveness* of testing.

A possible alternative or interim process for establishing the merit of PCA3 testing as an intervention might be a careful evaluation of the prognostic impact of the test, followed by an effort to establish a chain of evidence to support testing. There was vigorous discussion of formal modeling as a mechanism to replace the need for more formal short- or long-term trials, but concerns were raised about the assumptions that would need to be made. Missed tumors should exhibit the same or more indolent behavior than those identified by testing; the ability of testing to reduce biopsies or to detect clinically significant tumors should not be a result of confounding by demographic characteristics in patient subgroups (age, ethnic background, family history, etc.). Shorter-term studies similar to the REDUCE trial have already been used to study PCA3 performance,[18,19] but could be replicated or expanded to better understand how the test impacts outcomes. The suggestion was also made to piggyback PCA3 testing on current trials studying active surveillance, similar to the recent report by Tosoian,[5] but with more detail on outcomes (prostatectomy results) and longer term followup.

Table 6. Study design evaluations for PCA3 Research Need 3, Research Question 3.1: Does addition of PCA3 testing change long-term health outcomes in prostate screening?

Study Design Considerations	Randomized Clinical Trials	Prospective Cohort Study	Modeling
Description of design	Patients at risk for prostate cancer (initial or repeat biopsy) based on elevated tPSA and/or abnormal DRE or with positive biopsies are randomized to receive PCA3 in addition to standard testing or standard testing alone. Long-term outcomes, including morbidity, mortality and quality of life followed over 10 to 20 years.	Patients with and without prostate cancer identified in an intended use population and tracked according to PCA3 status --tested or not tested, positive or negative test results).Patients followed prospectively to determine choices about biopsy and treatment.	Estimates of outcomes would be made based on what is known about the natural history of prostate cancer and what is learned through the studies in Research Question 2.1 about likely behavior of cancers diagnosed or treated using information from PCA3 testing.
Advantages of study design for producing a valid result	The gold standard for understanding health care outcomes occurring as a result of use of PCA3 testing. Clinical characteristics can be carefully balanced.	Baseline characteristics can be measured, but may not be balanced. Statistical techniques may be able to partially control potential bias.	Modeling allows predictions of outcomes from use of PCA3 based on logical assumptions of tumor behavior and known impact of interventions. However, the strength of the model will depend on the reliability of the assumptions made. While it is possible that informed decisions will be made based on this modeling, the validity will not be well established. Technique has been used by the United States Preventive Services Task Force in developing some recommendations.
Resource use, size, and duration	This is likely to be a resource-intense process of large size, long duration, and high cost. Compliance may be a problem if diagnostic and therapeutic choices change during the duration of the study.	Resource use, size, and duration are likely to be similar to that of a randomized clinical trial. Compliance may be a problem if diagnostic and therapeutic choices change during the duration of the study.	Likely to be less resource-intense than other approaches.
Ethical, legal and social issues	Minimal; although the test has been approved by FDA for repeat biopsy (previous negative biopsy patients), there is no information on health care outcomes, hence the need for study.	Minimal; although the test has been approved by FDA for repeat biopsy (previous negative biopsy patients), there is no information on health care outcomes, hence the need for study.	None.
Availability of data or ability to recruit	Biopsy or treatment choice is commonly encountered in urological practice; the area is one of considerable physician and patient interest; recruitment would be expected to be relatively straightforward.	Biopsy or treatment choice is commonly encountered in urological practice; the area is one of considerable physician and patient interest; recruitment would be expected to be relatively straightforward.	This is an area of considerable interest to both physicians and statisticians; this would be a fertile area of collaboration.

Abbreviations: DRE = digital rectal examination FDA = U.S. Food and Drug Administration; PCA3 = prostate cancer antigen 3 gene; PSA = prostate-specific antigen; tPSA = total prostate-specific antigen

Discussion

Using the 2012 draft CER on PCA3 Testing in the Diagnosis and Management of Prostate Cancer, and with input from a diverse group of Stakeholders, a 10-step process was followed for identifying and prioritizing clinically important research needs and research questions. The research needs reflecting the breadth of the original CER Key Questions, included uncertainty about the diagnostic performance of PCA3, its ability to produce better biopsy or treatment decisions, and its impact on long-term health outcomes. The final research questions added specificity to these research needs. Through the process employed, a final list of three research needs and six associated research questions was compiled.

Given the complexity of topics discussed in the CER, the decision to limit the future research needs project to items within the clinical scope of testing, and to not address more general methodological and statistical issues, assured focus to the project. Although the CER did identify methodological problems that are worth addressing (including a general poor quality of the studies themselves), these are not unique to PCA3 and warrant further discussion in future projects, perhaps in the form of a series of methods papers.

There are several strengths to the process used to identify and prioritize research needs and research questions. First, the Stakeholders came from a wide variety of relevant disciplines, which was important to provide a balanced and broad perspective on the research needs being discussed. Second, the use of a variety of interactive communication approaches, including a one-on-one orientation to the project, two teleconferences, and the use of e-mails and internet surveys, allowed work to proceed in an efficient and timely manner. Third, there was active and vigorous participation by the Stakeholders in all phases of the project.

The Stakeholders agreed with the findings of the CER and recognized that work needed to be done to better understand the clinical performance, impact on decisionmaking, and health outcomes of PCA3 testing. Three stakeholders had previously served as Key Informants or members of the Technical Expert Panel for the PCA3 CER, and two had provided peer review of PCA3 CER document. The patient advocate was particularly helpful in calling attention to the patient's perspective on how important it would be to determine if PCA3 is viewed as a benefit, or as simply another confounding factor in the complex and difficult process of decisionmaking in at-risk patients.

In evaluating the prioritization of the research needs by the Stakeholders, a logical pattern evolved that seemed to fit well with the development and credentialing of a new diagnostic test. Highest priority went to establishing the diagnostic accuracy of the test. This is a highly pragmatic starting point, since without a clinically validated signal, risk of failure in further exploration of the use of a new test is high. Of second priority was defining what information the test signal conveyed about aggressiveness of missed or identified disease and how this information might be used in decisionmaking. It is likely that a test with a weak signal or that was poor at discriminating between indolent and aggressive disease might not convince physicians or patients, in either real or simulated studies, to make changes in management choices. The value of such a test would obviously be limited. Finally, in order to understand how a test impacts health outcomes, there is a need for either clinical studies or for a strong chain of evidence based on carefully selected and documented surrogates for predicting outcomes.

Because of the well-established hierarchal approach provided by the Stakeholders, the final rating of research questions was modified to rate questions within each research need rather than to generically evaluate these questions collectively across the research needs.

Recognizing the difficulty in performing the randomized clinical trial that would be required to establish the ultimate benefits and risks of testing, the Stakeholders provided the pragmatic direction of considering mechanisms for establishing how well PCA3 served as a prognostic marker of tumor aggressiveness. This association, if established strongly enough, was noted to be a potential measurement that could, by itself, convey value to testing by improving both diagnostic and treatment choices. Suggestions from the Stakeholders included use of prognostic features on biopsy, changes in grading between biopsy and prostatectomy, and add-on studies to ongoing investigations of active surveillance in carefully chosen patients.

Conclusions

This PCA3 FRN project was built from the PCA3 CER. A panel of Stakeholders refined and prioritized research needs and research questions. The results of this process are the following three top-ranked research needs and six research questions.

Research Need Number 1: Lack of information on the comparative performance of PCA3 and currently used biomarkers to detect prostate cancer; lack of "matched studies" on comparators.

- **Research Question 1.1:** What is the comparative effectiveness of PCA3 compared to the two commonly used add on tests of fPSA and tPSA velocity/doubling time in predicting prostate biopsy results?
- **Research Question 1.2:** What are PCA3's diagnostic performance characteristics in patients with elevated tPSA levels?
- **Research Question 1.3:** What is the comparative effectiveness of PCA3 compared to externally validated nomograms in predicting prostate biopsy results?

Research Need Number 2: Lack of studies on how PCA3 actually helps in biopsy or treatment decision making.

- **Research Question 2.1:** What information does PCA3 provide about the aggressiveness of prostate cancer? Do positive results correlate to tumors with aggressive features on biopsy or upgrading of tumors on prostatectomy? Do negative results correlate to tumors that may not require identification or aggressive treatment?
- **Research Question 2.2:** Does the addition of PCA3, either alone, or in combination with other markers, change prostate cancer biopsy or treatment decisionmaking for the patient or physician?

Research Need Number 3: Uncertainty of impact of PCA3 in biopsy decisionmaking on long term health outcomes.

- **Research Question 3.1:** Does addition of PCA3 testing change long term health outcomes in prostate screening?

References

1. Jemal A, Siegel R, Xu J, et al. Cancer statistics, 2010. CA Cancer J Clin. 2010 Sep-Oct;60(5):277-300. PMID: 20610543.

2. Freedland SJ. Screening, risk assessment, and the approach to therapy in patients with prostate cancer. Cancer. 2011 Mar 15;117(6):1123-35. PMID: 20960523.

3. Yin M, Bastacky S, Chandran U, et al. Prevalence of incidental prostate cancer in the general population: A study of healthy organ donors. J Urol. 2008 Mar;179(3):892-5; discussion 5. PMID: 18207193.

4. Sutcliffe P, Hummel S, Simpson E. Use of classical and novel biomarkers as prognostic risk factors for localised prostate cancer: A systematic review. Health Technol Assess. 2009;13:1-260.

5. Tosoian J, Loeb S. PSA and beyond: the past, present, and future of investigative biomarkers for prostate cancer. Scientific World J. 2010;10:1919-31. PMID: 20890581.

6. Moyer VA. Screening for Prostate Cancer: U.S. Preventive Services Task Force Recommendation Statement. Ann Intern Med. 2012 May 21PMID: 22615453.

7. Draisma G, Boer R, Otto SJ, et al. Lead times and overdetection due to prostate-specific antigen screening: estimates from the European Randomized Study of Screening for Prostate Cancer. J Natl Cancer Inst. 2003;95(12):868-78.

8. Bussemakers MJ, van Bokhoven A, Verhaegh GW, et al. DD3: a new prostate-specific gene, highly overexpressed in prostate cancer. Cancer Res. 1999 Dec 1;59(23):5975-9. PMID: 10606244.

9. Whitlock EP, Lopez SA, Chang S, et al. AHRQ Series Paper 3: Identifying, selecting, and refining topics for comparative effectiveness systematic reviews: AHRQ and the Effective Health-Care program. J Clin Epidemiol. 2010;63:491-501.

10. Robinson KA, Saldanha IJ, NA. M. Frameworks for determining research gaps during systematic reviews. Methods Future Research Needs Report No. 2. (Prepared by the Johns Hopkins University Evidence-based Practice Center under Contract No. HHSA 290-2007-10061-I.) AHRQ Publication No. 11-EHC043-EF. Rockville, MD: Agency for Healthcare Research and Quality. June 2011.

11. Carey T, Sanders G, Viswanathan M, et al. Framework for Considering Study Designs for Future Research Needs. Methods Future Research Needs Paper No. 8 (Prepared by the RTI–UNC Evidence-based Practice Center under Contract No. 290-2007-10056-I.) AHRQ Publication No. 12-EHC048-EF. Rockville, MD: Agency for Healthcare Research and Quality. March 2012. www.effectivehealthcare.ahrq.gov/reports/final.cfm.

12. Bossuyt PM, Reitsma JB, Bruns DE, et al. Towards complete and accurate reporting of studies of diagnostic accuracy: the STARD initiative. Standards for Reporting of Diagnostic Accuracy. Clin Chem. 2003 Jan;49(1):1-6. PMID: 12507953.

13. Bossuyt PM, Reitsma JB, Bruns DE, et al. The STARD statement for reporting studies of diagnostic accuracy: explanation and elaboration. Clin Chem. 2003 Jan;49(1):7-18. PMID: 12507954.

14. Simon RM, Paik S, Hayes DF. Use of archived specimens in evaluation of prognostic and predictive biomarkers. J Natl Cancer Inst. 2009;101(21):1446-52.

15. Coates RJ, Kolor K, Stewart SL, et al. Diagnostic markers for ovarian cancer screening: Not ready for routine clinical use. Clin Cancer Res. 2008;13:7575.

16. Visintin I, Feng Z, Longton G, et al. Diagnostic markers for early detection of ovarian cancer. Clin Cancer Res. 2008 Feb 15;14(4):1065-72. PMID: 18258665.

17. Mauger B, Rothenberg B, Marbella A, et al. Future Research Needs for Comparataive Effectiveness of Treatments for Localized Prostate Cancer. Future Research Needs Paper No. 4 (Prepared by Blue Cross and Blue Shield Association, Technology Evaluation Center Evidence-based Practice Center under contract No. 290-2007-10058-1). AHRQ Publication No. 10-EHC072-EF. Rockville, MD: Agency for Healthcare Research: September 2010. www.effectivehealthcare.ahrq.gov/reports/final.cfm.

18. Aubin SM, Reid J, Sarno MJ, et al. PCA3 molecular urine test for predicting repeat prostate biopsy outcome in populations at risk: Validation in the placebo arm of the dutasteride REDUCE trial. J Urol. 2010 Nov;184(5):1947-52. PMID: 20850153.

19. Aubin SM, Reid J, Sarno MJ, et al. Prostate cancer gene 3 score predicts prostate biopsy outcome in men receiving dutasteride for prevention of prostate cancer: results from the REDUCE trial. Urology. 2011 Aug;78(2):380-5. PMID: 21820580.

20. Cooperberg MR, Carroll PR, Klotz L. Active surveillance for prostate cancer: progress and promise. J Clin Oncol. 2011;29:3669-76.

Appendix A. Conclusions From Draft Comparative Effectiveness Review of PCA3 for Detection and Treatment of Prostate Cancer

Key Questions 1 and 2: Testing PCA3 and Comparators To Identify Men With Prostate Cancer in Initial or Repeat Biopsies

Results and Strength of Evidence of PCA3 by Biopsy Status

Data was insufficient to evaluate PCA3 performance for key question 1 or 2 alone. Analysis of comparative matched PCA3:tPSA AUC curves and of performance at a pre-set PCA3 specificity of 50% indicated PCA3 performance did not appear to be affected by the biopsy status of patients. Therefore studies were combined and used to answer Key Questions 1 and 2 together.

Results and Strength of Evidence of Comparison of PCA3 to tPSA

With regard to diagnostic accuracy, PCA3 was more discriminatory for detecting prostate cancer than extent of tPSA elevations. At any set clinical sensitivity, the clinical specificity of PCA3 testing is higher than that of tPSA. In addition, at any set clinical specificity, the clinical sensitivity of PCA3 was higher than that of tPSA. These two biomarkers appeared to be independent in detection of prostate. The strength of evidence for diagnostic accuracy was *low*.

With regard to the intermediate outcome of improved decisionmaking, PCA3 does have the potential to reduce unnecessary biopsies when compared to tPSA alone, by increasing the detection of true negative results and reducing potential harms of false positive results. However, no studies were identified that reported on this outcome. In addition, no studies were identified that addressed long-term outcomes (e.g., mortality, morbidity, quality of life) related to PCA3 and tPSA testing. The strength of evidence for these outcomes was *insufficient*.

Results and Strength of Evidence of Comparison of PCA3 to Other Comparators

The data were missing or inadequate for comparison of PCA3 testing to the other selected biomarkers with regard to intermediate and long-term outcomes. The strength of evidence for all comparators was *insufficient*.

Key Question 3: Testing PCA3 and Comparators To Identify Low Risk/Indolent Patients Who May Be Candidates for Active Surveillance

Results and Strength of Evidence of PCA3 to Other Comparators

Estimation of diagnostic accuracy and assessment of intermediate outcomes (e.g., impact on decisionmaking and/or treatment harms) requires the use of a reference or gold standard. In this intended use, that would require a more long-term clinical endpoint or endpoints (e.g., measures of progression, metastasis, prostate cancer related morbidity), or a validated surrogate. Seven prospective studies of cohorts of men in active surveillance are currently ongoing. The one partially informative study in this review came from one of these groups. Median followup in these studies ranges from only two to seven years, so short term outcomes collected included percent progressing (i.e., increased grade/volume or PSA/PSA velocity) and time to progression.

More time will be needed for assessment of progression-free survival.[20] Consequently, it is not surprising that no studies were identified that provided outcome information to support estimation of diagnostic accuracy or clinical impact of testing with PCA3 or comparators. The strength of evidence for all comparators and outcomes was *insufficient*.

Appendix B. Methodological and Statistical Gaps in Knowledge About PCA3 Testing

Key Questions 1 and 2

1. What modeling approach/algorithm would allow for the easiest inclusion of new markers while reducing the need for independent verification? Most reported multivariate modeling of prostate cancer risk relies on logistic regression. These models are difficult to compare across studies and do not allow for simple inclusion of new variables without re-computing all coefficients. Other models, such as multivariate overlapping Gaussian distributions, may fit the markers of interest and might allow for easier comparisons as well as the ability to easily add (or subtract) markers as knowledge increases. This could also allow for validation of partial models, if some markers have not been measured.

2. What factors influence whether partial verification bias impacts the tPSA and/or the matched tPSA/PCA3 ROC curves? Factors that could be explored include the range of cancer rates, the range of verification rates, and the use of continuous versus categorical verification corrections. There have been only a handful of reports on tPSA use that address partial verification bias. A better understanding of this issue is needed if PCA3 is to be properly evaluated in the context of the widespread use of tPSA as triage test for treatment decisions.

3. What absolute cut-offs or continuous values can be assigned to the PCA3 assay across the ROC curve? While the analyses in this review provide an approximate ROC curve allowing interpolation of sensitivity and false positive rates across the range of values, the absolute PCA3 and tPSA cut-offs may not be appropriate in every setting.

4. Does our review's literature restriction to matched studies provide more consistent and reliable comparisons than had the review used independent summaries of each marker's performance? Given the increasing emphasis on comparative effectiveness analyses, a formal comparison of these two methods might provide useful guidance to future reviews.

5. Does the reporting of matched analyses improve the usefulness of the dataset? Although our inclusion criteria required PCA3 and a comparator to be measured in the same population, it did not require a formal matched analysis to be reported. Thus, the reports did not allow for a comparison of how many men with cancer were identified by both markers, neither of the markers, or only one or the other marker. Requesting such analyses be performed using existing datasets would help answer this question.

6. How can researchers studying PCA3 and other comparators be encouraged to provide proper reporting of statistical details? Proper reporting of statistical information on studies of PCA3 and the comparators was often absent in articles evaluated for this review. These include: confidence intervals, standard errors, prediction limits and other measure of dispersion and precision for all effect measures as well as good summary parameters for their data (e.g., selected centiles, medians, geometric means and trimmed logarithmic standard deviations). All studies identified were of poor quality when rated by QUADAS.

7. How can systematic differences in marker levels due to reagents/manufactures be minimized or accounted for by analysis? Systematic differences between reagents/manufacturers exist for at least some of the markers that can influence the tests performance at fixed mass unit cut-offs.

Key Question 3

1. Can intermediate outcomes, such as cancer classifications of aggressive or indolent tumors be properly validated? Given that current clinical practice guidelines employ unvalidated, or partially validated intermediate outcomes, it is difficult to design studies that would provide proper validation. Exploration of what study designs or re-analyses of existing dataset might provide stronger validation of select intermediate measures could be undertaken.

2. What is the impact of use of PCA3 on long-term health outcomes when used to help select patients for active surveillance versus aggressive treatment?

Appendix C. Search Strategy for Recently Published and Ongoing Studies on PCA3 Testing

PUBMED on 5/15/2012
("prostate cancer antigen 3, human" [Supplementary Concept] OR "PCA3" OR "DD3" OR "DD3PCA3" OR "DD3(PCA3)" OR "prostate cancer gene 3" OR "prostate cancer antigen 3" OR "progensa" OR "differential display code 3") AND ("prostate" OR "prostatic")
Limits: English, Dates 8/1/2011 to 5/15/2012

Results: 31 citations

EMBASE.COM on 5/15/2012
'prostate cancer antigen 3, human' OR pca3 OR dd3 OR dd3pca3 OR 'dd3(pca3)' OR 'prostate cancer gene 3' OR 'prostate cancer antigen 3' OR progensa OR 'differential display code 3' AND ('prostate'/exp OR prostatic)
Limits: English, Dates 8/1/2011 to 5/15/2012

Results: 76 citations

Cochrane Central on 5/15/2012
prostate cancer antigen 3 OR pca3 OR dd3 OR dd3pca3 OR dd3(pca3) OR prostate cancer gene 3 OR prostate cancer antigen 3 OR progensa OR differential display code 3' AND ('prostate'/exp OR prostatic)

Results: No new trials identified

Clinical Trials.Gov
prostate cancer antigen 3 OR pca3 OR dd3 OR dd3pca3 OR dd3(pca3) OR prostate cancer gene 3 OR prostate cancer antigen 3 OR progensa

Results: 3 Newly updated trial records

ASCO
prostate cancer antigen 3 OR pca3 OR dd3 OR dd3pca3 OR dd3(pca3) OR prostate cancer gene 3 OR prostate cancer antigen 3 OR progensa

Results: 3 2012 ASCO Conference Abstracts

Appendix D. Literature Relevant to PCA3 Research Needs

Key Question 1 and 2: In patients with elevated PSA and/or abnormal DRE who are candidates for biopsy or repeat biopsy what is the comparative effectiveness of PCA3 testing as a replacement for or addition to standard tests?

Table D.1. Literature relevant to Key Questions 1 and 2

Broad Research Needs	Specific Research Needs	Comments from Stakeholders	Primary Studies	Abstracts (published since CER)	Ongoing Clinical Trials
Diagnostic accuracy of PCA3	1. Lack of information on the comparative performance of PCA3 and currently used biomarkers to detect prostate cancer; lack of "matched studies" on comparators 2. Lack of a definition of "clinically significant improvement" in diagnostic accuracy. 3. Potential for comparisons of PCA3 with tPSA to be affected by inadequate clinical characterization of populations studied 4. Lack of information on how demographics impact PCA3 test	Defining diagnostic accuracy is critical to test use; matched studies are needed Consider reaching out to researchers to better synthesize what information is now available Having a target for accuracy is important – a question to answer is how accurate is accurate enough Biopsy is not a perfect gold standard; consider use in context of imaging. Biopsy is not perfect; consider using prostatectomy outcomes to better understand what kinds of tumors are being detected	**From CER:** Adam 2011 Ankerst 2008 Aubin 2010 de la Taille 2011 Deras 2008 FDA 2012 Haese 2008 Hessels 2010 Mearini 2009 Nyberg 2010 Ochiai 2011 Ouyang 2009 Perdona 2011 Rigau M 2010 Roobol 2010 Schilling 2010 Wang 2009 **Updated Literature Search** Auprich 2011 Bollito 2012 Ferro 2012 Goode 2012 Pepe 2012 Wu 2012	Urinary PCA3 as a predictor for prostate cancer in a cohort of 1928 men undergoing initial prostate biopsy, Chevli et al., American Urological Association, May 21, 2012 PROGENSA PCA3 pivotal U.S. clinical study confirms utility for predicting repeat biopsy outcome. Ward et al., American Urological Association, May 21, 2012 The NCI Early Detection Research Network (EDRN) urinary PCA3 validation trial, Wei et al., American Urological Association, May 23, 2012 PCA3 test as an adjunct in diagnosis of prostate cancer, Yutkin et al., American Urological Association, May 23, 2012	NCT01177426, Prostate Cancer Antigen 3 (PCA-3) Gene Project – recruiting NCT01441687, Expressed Prostatic Secretion and Post Massage Urine Biomarkers in Predicting Biopsy Results in Patients Undergoing Prostate Biopsy -- recruiting

Broad Research Needs	Specific Research Needs	Comments from Stakeholders	Primary Studies	Abstracts (published since CER)	Ongoing Clinical Trials
Use of PCA3 in Biopsy Decisionmaking	5. Lack of information on the impact of PCA3 on short term outcomes such as biopsy decisionmaking	Might adjust analytical framework to emphasize desired outcome; decreased biopsies and less overtreatment Consider modeling using what is known about cancer detection to determine the impact of avoiding biopsies Consider how this might relate to current use of imaging technologies	None identified	The appropriateness of active surveillance and the impact of prostate cancer gene 3 (PCA3) in low risk prostate cancer: an analysis of expert opinion, Speakman et al. Urology, 2011 79(3):S320	None identified
Effect of PCA3 on long-term health outcomes	6. Uncertainty of impact of PCA3 on long-term health outcomes	Needed but how practical; morbidity is already low, PCA3 might have a hard time proving its merits Evaluation of testing should be performed with attention to what is known or not known about value of PSA screening itself and the fact this matter may have not been settled	None identified	None identified	None identified

Key Question 3: In patients with positive prostate biopsies what is the comparative effectiveness of PCA3 testing as a replacement for or addition to standard tests in treatment decisionmaking (active surveillance versus more aggressive therapy)?

Table D.2. Literature relevant to Key Question 3

Research Need	CER Findings	Stakeholders	Primary Studies	Abstracts (published since CER)	Ongoing Clinical Trials
Diagnostic accuracy of PCA3	7. Lack of clear endpoint to establish performance; when PCA3 disagrees with other inclusion criteria; how do you know which is right?	No comments	**From CER:** Liss 2011 Nakanishi 2008 Ploussard 2011 Vlaeminck-Guillem 2011 Whitman 2008 **Updated Lit Search** Durand 2012 Van Poppel 2011	Longitudinal followup of prostate specific antigen (PSA) and prostate cancer antigen-3 (PCA3 in men with stable disease on active surveillance, Dangle et al., American Urological Association, May 22, 2012	None identified
Use of PCA3 in Treatment Decisionmaking	8. Lack of studies on how PCA3 actually helps in treatment decisionmaking?	Possible role as a prognostic marker and in making refinements in therapy beyond active surveillance and aggressive therapy	None identified	None identified	None identified
Effect of PCA3 on Long-term Health Outcomes	9. Lack of information on the impact of PCA3 on long-term health outcomes	No comments	None Identified	None identified	None identified

References for Primary Studies

References for Primary Studies

1. Adam A, Engelbrecht MJ, Bornman MS, et al. The role of the PCA3 assay in predicting prostate biopsy outcome in a South African setting. BJU Int. 2011 Apr 20; PMID: 21507188.

2. Ankerst DP, Groskopf J, Day JR, et al. Predicting prostate cancer risk through incorporation of prostate cancer gene 3. J Urol. 2008 Oct;180(4):1303-8; discussion 08. PMID: 18707724.

3. Aubin SM, Reid J, Sarno MJ, et al. PCA3 molecular urine test for predicting repeat prostate biopsy outcome in populations at risk: validation in the placebo arm of the dutasteride REDUCE trial. J Urol. 2010 Nov;184(5):1947-52. PMID: 20850153.

4. Auprich M, Haese A, Walz J et al. External validation of urinary PCA3-based nomograms to individually predict prostate biopsy outcome. Eur Urol. 2010; 58(5):727-32. PMID: 21939492

5. Bollito E, De Luca S, Cicilano M, et al. Prostate cancer gene 3 urine assay cutoff in diagnosis of prostate cancer: A validation study on an Italian patient population undergoing first and repeat biopsy. Anal Quant Cytol Histol. 2012 Apr;34(2):96-104.

6. de la Taille A, Irani J, Graefen M, et al. Clinical evaluation of the PCA3 assay in guiding initial biopsy decisions. J Urol. 2011 Jun;185(6):2119-25. PMID: 21496856.

7. Deras IL, Aubin SM, Blase A, et al. PCA3: a molecular urine assay for predicting prostate biopsy outcome. J Urol. 2008 Apr;179(4):1587-92. PMID: 18295257.

8. Durand X, Xylinas E, Radulescu C et al. The value of urinary prostate cancer gene 3 (PCA3) scores in predicting pathological features at radical prostatectomy. BJU Int. 2012; 110(1):43-9. PMID: 22221521

9. FDA Summary of Safety and Effectiveness – Progensa PCA3. www.accessdata.fda.gov/cdrh_docs/pdf10/P100033b.pdf

10. Ferro M, Bruzzese D, Perdona S et al. Predicting prostate biopsy outcome: prostate health index (phi) and prostate cancer antigen 3 (PCA3) are useful biomarkers. *Clinica chimica acta*; Int J Clin Chem. 2012; 413(15-16):1274-8. PMID: 22542564

11. Goode RR, Marshall SJ, Duff M et al. Use of PCA3 in detecting prostate cancer in initial and repeat prostate biopsy patients. Prostate. 2012. PMID: 22585386

12. Haese A, de la Taille A, van Poppel H, et al., Clinical utility of the PCA3 urine assay in European men scheduled for repeat biopsy. Eur Urol. 2008 Nov; 54(5):1081-8. PMID: 18602209

13. Hessels D, van Gils MP, van Hooij O, et al. Predictive value of PCA3 in urinary sediments in determining clinico-pathological characteristics of prostate cancer. Prostate. 2010 Jan 1;70(1):10-6. PMID: 19708043.

14. Liss MA, Santos R, Osann K, et al. PCA3 molecular urine assay for prostate cancer: association with pathologic features and impact of collection protocols. World J Urol. 2011 Oct;29(5):683-8. PMID: 2115292.

15. Mearini E, Antognelli C, Del Buono C, et al. The combination of urine DD3(PCA3) mRNA and PSA mRNA as molecular markers of prostate cancer. Biomarkers. 2009 Jun;14(4):235-43. PMID: 19489685.

16. Nakanishi H, Groskopf J, Fritsche HA, et al. PCA3 molecular urine assay correlates with prostate cancer tumor volume: implication in selecting candidates for active surveillance. J Urol. 2008 May;179(5):1804-9; discussion 09-10. PMID: 18353398.

17. Nyberg M, Ulmert D, Lindgren A, et al. PCA3 as a diagnostic marker for prostate cancer: a validation study on a Swedish patient population. Scand J Urol Nephrol. 2010 Dec;44(6):378-83. PMID: 20961267.

18. Ochiai A, Okihara K, Kamoi K, et al. Prostate cancer gene 3 urine assay for prostate cancer in Japanese men undergoing prostate biopsy. Int J Urol. 2011 Mar;18(3):200-5. PMID: 21332814.

19. Ouyang B, Bracken B, Burke B, et al. A duplex quantitative polymerase chain reaction assay based on quantification of alpha-methylacyl-CoA racemase transcripts and prostate cancer antigen 3 in urine sediments improved diagnostic accuracy for prostate cancer. J Urol. 2009 Jun;181(6):2508-13; discussion 13-4. PMID: 19371911.

20. Pepe P, Fraggetta F, Galia A, Aragona F. Is PCA3 score useful in preoperative staging of a single microfocus of prostate cancer diagnosed at saturation biopsy? Urol Int. 2012 Aug 3. [Epub ahead of print].

21. Perdona S, Cavadas V, Di Lorenzo G, et al. Prostate cancer detection in the "grey area" of prostate-specific antigen below 10 ng/ml: head-to-head comparison of the updated PCPT calculator and Chun's nomogram, two risk estimators incorporating prostate cancer antigen 3. Eur Urol. 2011 Jan;59(1):81-7. PMID: 20947244.

22. Ploussard G, Durand X, Xylinas E, et al. Prostate cancer antigen 3 score accurately predicts tumour volume and might help in selecting prostate cancer patients for active surveillance. Eur Urol. 2011 Mar;59(3):422-9, PMID: 21156337.

23. Rigau M, Morote J, Mir MC, et al. PSGR and PCA3 as biomarkers for the detection of prostate cancer in urine. Prostate. 2010 Dec 1;70(16):1760-7. PMID: 20672322.

24. Roobol MJ, Schroder FH, van Leeuwen P, et al. Performance of the prostate cancer antigen 3 (PCA3) gene and prostate-specific antigen in prescreened men: exploring the value of PCA3 for a first-line diagnostic test. Eur Urol. 2010 Oct;58(4):475-81. PMID: 20637539.

25. Schilling D, Hennenlotter J, Munz M, et al. Interpretation of the prostate cancer gene 3 in reference to the individual clinical background: implications for daily practice. Urol Int. 2010 85(2):159-65. PMID: 20424427.

26. Vlaeminck-Guillem V, Devonec M, Colombel M, et al. Urinary PCA3 score predicts prostate cancer multifocality. J Urol. 2011 Apr;185(4):1234-9. PMID: 21334023

27. Van Poppel, Haese, Graefen et al. The relationship between Proostate Cancer gene 3 (PCA3) and prostate cancer significance. BJU Int. 2011 Aug 26;109:360-366. PMID: 21883822

28. Wang R, Chinnaiyan AM, Dunn RL, et al. Rational approach to implementation of prostate cancer antigen 3 into clinical care. Cancer. 2009 Sep 1;115(17):3879-86. PMID: 19517474.

29. Whitman EJ, Groskopf J, Ali A, et al. PCA3 score before radical prostatectomy predicts extracapsular extension and tumor volume. J Urol. 2008 Nov;180(5):1975-8; discussion 78-9. PMID: 18801539.

30. Wu AK, Reese AC, Cooperberg MR et al. Utility of PCA3 in patients undergoing repeat biopsy for prostate cancer. Prostate Cancer and Prostatic Dis. 2012; 15(1):100-5. PMID: 22042252.

Appendix E. SurveyMonkey® Form for Prioritizing PCA3 Research Needs

Please rank your top 3 research needs from 1 to 3, with 3 having the highest priority and 1 the lowest.

1. Lack of information on the comparative performance of PCA3 and currently used biomarkers to detect prostate cancer; lack of "matched studies" on comparators.

2. Lack of a definition of "clinically significant improvement" in diagnostic accuracy.

3. Potential for comparisons of PCA3 with tPSA to be affected by inadequate clinical characterization of populations studied (e.g., verification bias).

4. Lack of information on how demographics impact PCA3 test.

5. Lack of information on the impact of PCA3 on short term outcomes such as biopsy decisionmaking.

6. Uncertainty of impact of PCA3 in biopsy decisionmaking on long term health outcomes.

7. Lack of clear endpoint to establish performance; when PCA3 disagrees with other inclusion criteria; how do you know which is right?

8. Lack of studies on how PCA3 actually helps in treatment decisionmaking.

9. Lack of information on the impact of PCA3 in treatment decisionmaking on long-term health outcomes.

Appendix F. Results From PCA3 Research Needs Prioritization Survey

Table F.1. Results from PCA3 future research needs prioritization survey

Rank	Research need	Total votes	Total Score
1	Lack of information on the comparative performance of PCA3 and currently used biomarkers to detect prostate cancer; lack of "matched studies" on comparators	4	11
2	Lack of studies on how PCA3 actually helps in treatment decisionmaking	4	8
3	Lack of information on the impact of PCA3 on short term outcomes such as biopsy decisionmaking	4	7
4	Uncertainty of impact of PCA3 in biopsy decisionmaking on long-term health outcomes	3	6
5	Lack of a definition of "clinically significant improvement" in diagnostic accuracy	2	5
6	Potential for comparisons of PCA3 with tPSA to be affected by inadequate clinical characterization of populations studied (e.g. verification bias)	3	4
6	Lack of clear endpoint to establish performance; when PCA3 disagrees with other inclusion criteria how do you know which is right?	2	4
7	Lack of information on the impact of PCA3 in treatment decisionmaking on long-term health outcomes	2	3
8	Lack of information on how demographics impact PCA3 test	0	0

Appendix G. SurveyMonkey® Form for Prioritizing PCA3 Research Questions

Research Need 1. Please rank your top three research questions from 1 to 3, with 3 having the highest priority and 1 the lowest.

1. What is the PCA3's diagnostic performance characteristics in patients with elevated tPSA levels?

2. What is the comparative effectiveness of PCA3 compared to the two commonly used add-on tests of fPSA and tPSA velocity/doubling time in predicting prostate biopsy results?

3. What is the comparative effectiveness of PCA3 compared to externally validated nomograms in predicting prostate biopsy results?

4. What is the comparative effectiveness of PCA3 compared to addition of PCA3 to externally validated nomograms in predicting prostate biopsy results?

Research Need 2. Please rank your top two research questions from 1 to 2, with 2 having the highest priority and 1 the lowest.

1. What information does PCA3 provide about the aggressiveness of prostate cancer? In other words, do positive results correlate to tumors with aggressive features on biopsy or upgrading of tumors on prostatectomy, and do negative results correlate to tumors that may not require identification or aggressive treatment?

2. Does the addition of PCA3, either alone or in combination with other markers, change prostate cancer biopsy or treatment decisionmaking for the patient or physician?

Appendix H. Results From PCA3 Research Questions Prioritization Survey

Table H.1. Results from PCA3 research needs prioritization survey

Rank	Research Need	Research Questions	Total Votes	Total Score
1	1. Lack of information on the comparative performance of PCA3 and currently used biomarkers to detect prostate cancer; lack of "matched studies" on comparators	What is the comparative effectiveness of PCA3 compared to the two commonly used add-on tests of fPSA and tPSA velocity/doubling time in predicting prostate biopsy results?	8	16
2		What are the PCA3's diagnostic performance characteristics in patients with elevated tPSA levels?	7	15
3		What is the comparative effectiveness of PCA3 compared to externally validated nomograms in predicting prostate biopsy results?	5	12
4		What is the comparative effectiveness of PCA3 compared to addition of PCA3 to externally validated nomograms in predicting prostate biopsy results?	4	5
1	2. Lack of studies on how PCA3 actually helps in biopsy or treatment decisionmaking	Does the addition of PCA3, either alone or in combination with other markers, change prostate cancer biopsy or treatment decisionmaking for the patient or physician?	8	12
1		What information does PCA3 provide about the aggressiveness of prostate cancer? In other words, do positive results correlate to tumors with aggressive features on biopsy or upgrading of tumors on prostatectomy, and do negative results correlate to tumors that may not require identification or aggressive treatment?	8	12

H-1

www.ingramcontent.com/pod-product-compliance
Lightning Source LLC
Chambersburg PA
CBHW081616170526

45166CB00009B/2988